OPEN

**why asking for help
can save your life**

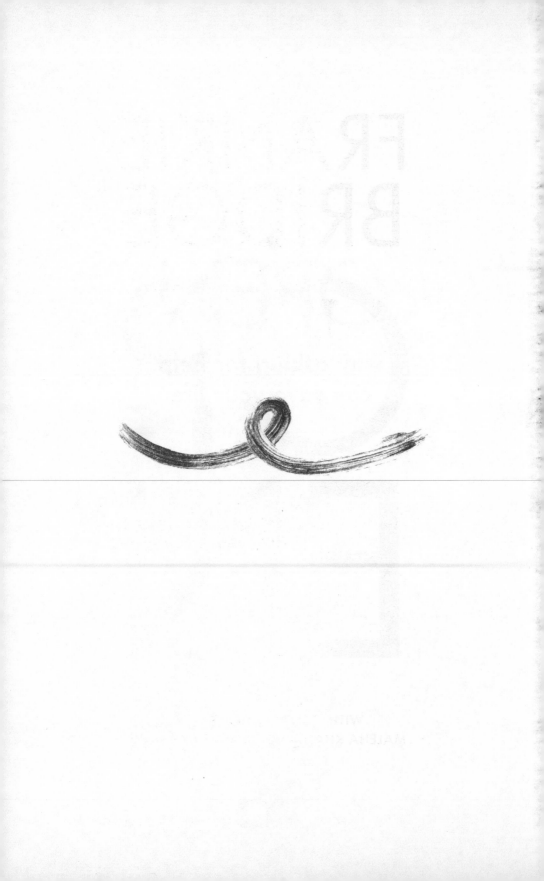

FRANKIE BRIDGE

OP EN

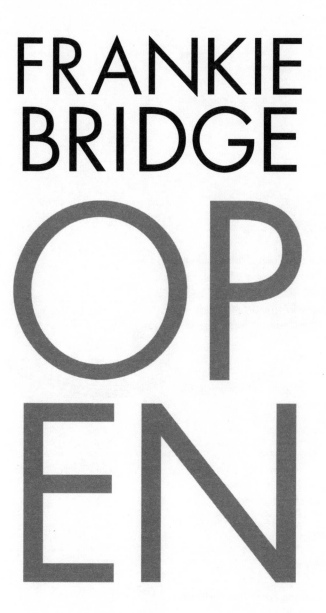

WITH CONTRIBUTIONS FROM
MALEHA KHAN AND DR MIKE MCPHILLIPS

An Hachette UK Company
www.hachette.co.uk

First published in Great Britain in 2020
by Cassell,
a division of Octopus Publishing Group Ltd
Carmelite House
50 Victoria Embankment
London EC4Y 0DZ
www.octopusbooks.co.uk

ISBN 978 1 78840 170 8

A CIP catalogue record for this book is
available from the British Library

Printed and bound in the UK

10 9 8 7 6 5 4 3

Senior Commissioning Editor: Romilly Morgan
Senior Editor: Alex Stetter
Additional text: Maleha Khan, Dr Mike
    McPhillips
Designer: Jack Storey
Senior Designer: Jaz Bahra
Cover Design: Two Associates
Author photographs: Sophie Davidson
Illustrations: Ella McLean
Production Controller: Grace O'Byrne

To you...

to help you on your way.

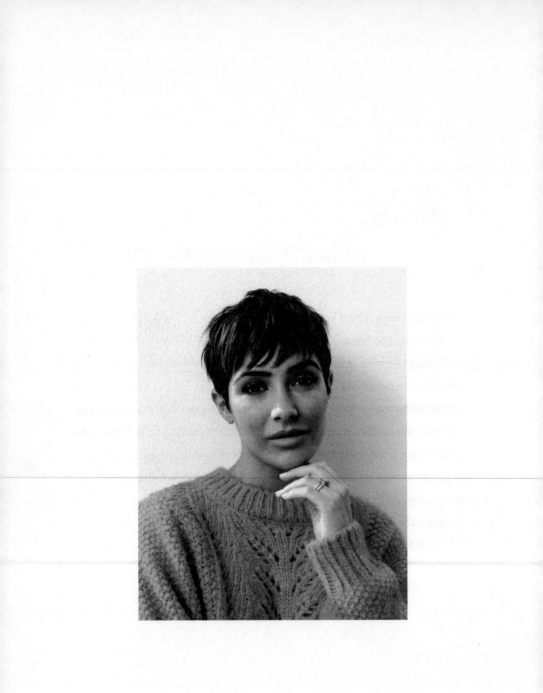

ABOUT THE AUTHOR

Frankie Bridge is best known as one-fifth of The Saturdays and outside of music, she has established herself as a TV presenter and digital influencer. Frankie became an ambassador for MIND after opening up about her experiences of anxiety, depression and panic attacks after her hospitalization in May 2012. Having initially dealt with these issues in silence, she has been keen to support MIND in making sure that no one has to face a mental health problem alone. Recently, Frankie has been a key player in helping to launch the MIND partnership with the mental health initiative Heads Together, as well as lending her support to Time to Talk Day. In 2019, she launched her first podcast series, OPEN MIND, focusing on mental health. It debuted in the top ten podcasts upon release.

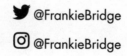

🐦 @FrankieBridge

📷 @FrankieBridge

CONTENTS

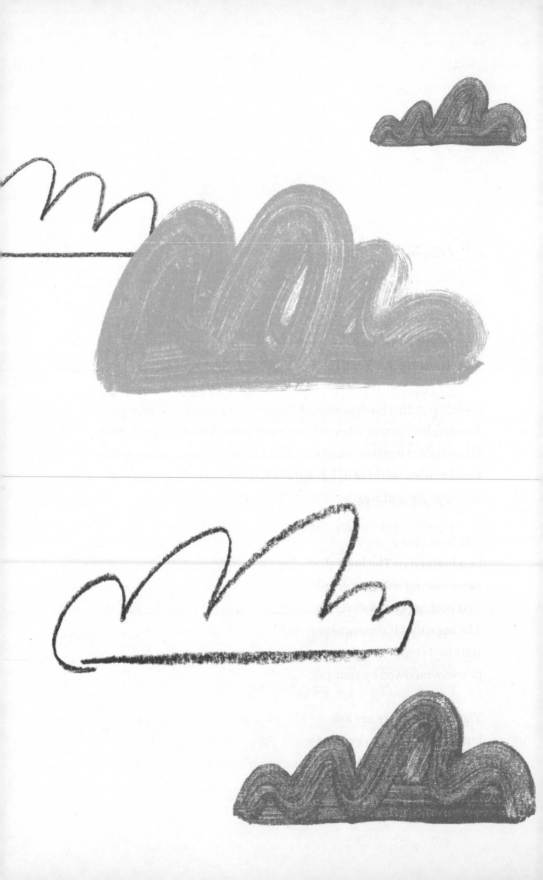

Dear You

I've tried to write this letter to you several times, but each time
I tried to begin I struggled to find the 'right' words. But recently
I realized that finding the right words, in the right order, at the
right time, is not what this book is about.

Simply put, this book is about finding and keeping hold of hope.
Because let's face it, when it comes to mental health, hope is often
all we have. Your own mental health battles or those of others can
make you lose sight of it, but hope is truly the one thing that will
keep you going through some of the harder times.

The hope that every day is a new day and that tomorrow could
be a better day. The hope that what you are currently feeling and
experiencing will pass sooner or later. Remembering to stay hopeful
that nothing lasts forever, including great sadness and happiness.
The hope that if you speak out and ask for help, you will be taking
your first steps towards ensuring that your future will not always
be overshadowed by your present.

The truth is, there are lots of things I wish I had told my former self,
but most of all it's to keep up hope. The Frankie I was when I was
unwell isn't the Frankie I am now, largely because I found my voice

to speak out and ask for help. But there are many hopeful and helpful things I wish I had told myself when I was suffering that I want to share with you before we go on this journey together, so that you too can find and hold onto hope through the bad times and the good:

Your life is still worth living and your future is brighter than you think. Yes, the dark clouds and the showers will come and sometimes the rain will fall hard without respite for a long time. There will be times when you feel as though it will flood every part of your body and mind and that you will drown because there is no way out. But the sunshine will always reappear, and some days will be brighter and warmer than ever before. Every time you step back into the light, you will grow stronger.

This too will pass. You will not feel this way forever and there will be a moment, although I can't say exactly when, when the clouds will clear and the sun will come out again. You need to give these brighter days as much of your emotion and your attention as the darker days.

You don't *need* to be fixed and you actually may never be fixed. What human is perfect or normal, anyway? Instead you just need to *accept* and learn how to live with how and who you are.

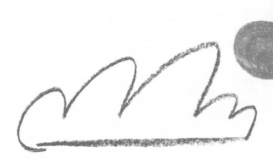

Don't try to push down overwhelming thoughts and feelings.
It will only make you feel more trapped and cut off from the world.
Take the time to learn about your condition and why you feel the
way you do. Understanding this will make it much easier to cope
when you're overwhelmed by your feelings, because you will have
an explanation for what is actually going on inside you and why it's
happening, rather than trying to control it, react to it or hide away
from it.

Give your feelings a name that makes sense to you. I call mine
my 'Sunshine and Showers', which serves to remind me that both
states exist within me and one will follow the other.

No one else is in charge of your happiness. Other people can
make things easier or they can make them harder, but finding
true happiness, deep within, is down to you.

There isn't going to be one thing that makes this all go away.
It won't be a career goal you reach, or a material possession you own,
or a defining moment in your personal life that will transform you
forever. Although these things may give you temporary happiness
and relief, it won't last as long as you need it to. The change has to
come from within you, rather than from the outside.

Nothing is coming around the corner to save you. You don't need saving, you can save yourself (with the help of friends and family, therapy, medication and whatever else may help make every day that bit easier).

There isn't always a specific reason for your unhappiness. Seek any help you can, go to the doctor, start therapy as soon as possible and take medication if that's what you need. The important thing is to give yourself every chance to get better before you try to fix everything *except* your mind.

Retraining your mind will be hard, but proving your instincts and automatic reactions wrong can become your superpower. Facing up to anxieties, insecurities and fears, taking them on and interrogating them is so empowering. These thoughts are often not based on reality or on what is actually happening around you, so learning how to stop letting them control you will help you to transform and reprogramme your mind into providing kinder, more supportive thoughts.

Even so, there will still be some days when breathing seems like too much of an effort. And there will also still be some days when just getting out of bed will be a huge accomplishment. Remember not to be down on yourself and to celebrate those small victories and be proud of overcoming whatever hurdle (large or small) that is placed in your way.

As hard as you find it to believe, people are not better off without you. There is still so much purpose left in your life. You are not crazy, you are not alone, you are *needed*, you are *loved* and you *matter*. The future is yours for the taking and living.

You are doing the best you can and that's pretty blooming awesome!

Frankie
x

Understanding
is key to
not being
afraid of
how you feel.

HOW THIS BOOK WORKS

Welcome to *Open*, in which I will take you through my journey with my mental health. It is an honest, personal account of what it's like to live with a mental illness and keep on surviving. I don't have the medical answers to help you deal with your illness, but I will share my own journey. I am a constant work in progress and every day I need something different to get me through.

My psychologist Mal Khan and my psychiatrist Mike McPhillips have helped me back onto the path of better health by giving me the tools and knowledge I need to better understand, manage and accept my illness. You will find comments from them about my symptoms and the various therapies I have tried, along with explanations not only of the different mental health issues I live with, but also the drivers behind them and the effects they have on me and those around me, throughout these pages. Their contributions aren't 'top tips' – if only treating mental illness was that easy – but I hope they will help you to understand what really happens behind the catch-all labels 'depression', 'anxiety' and 'panic'. Because understanding is key to not being afraid of how you feel.

So, here it is, my story about the really tough side of mental health that no one talks about. This is what it is like living a life with an illness, an invisible illness that there's still so much more to learn about and to understand and which can hit at any point in a person's life, regardless of who they are, what they have, or whether they are strong or weak characters. One that has been ignored and not understood for so many years and that, only now, is starting to be recognized. Something for which there is no rule book and no perfect solution.

I want to let you know that you are not alone. We can all help, and be helped, because we're all in this together.

The truth is, it affects most of us.

Clinical psychologists generally have a first degree in psychology and further doctoral training in clinical psychology. They specialize in the diagnosis and psychological treatment of mental, behavioural and emotional illnesses. They do not prescribe medications (although they might recommend that a client needs medication), but use a range of psychological techniques such as Cognitive Behavioural Therapy (CBT).

Psychiatrists are fully trained doctors who have specialized in psychiatry. They can make a medical diagnosis of mental disorders, prescribe medications such as antidepressants, sedatives and antipsychotics, prescribe physical treatments like electoconvulsive therapy (ECT), admit people to psychiatric hospital, detain people involuntarily for their own protection or the protection of others (known as 'sectioning'), and refer patients for various talking therapies.

In this book, you will find contributions from my psychologist Mal Khan and my psychiatrist Dr Mike McPhillips. Their comments are marked with the symbols below:

MALEHA KHAN
psychologist

DR MIKE McPHILLIPS
psychiatrist

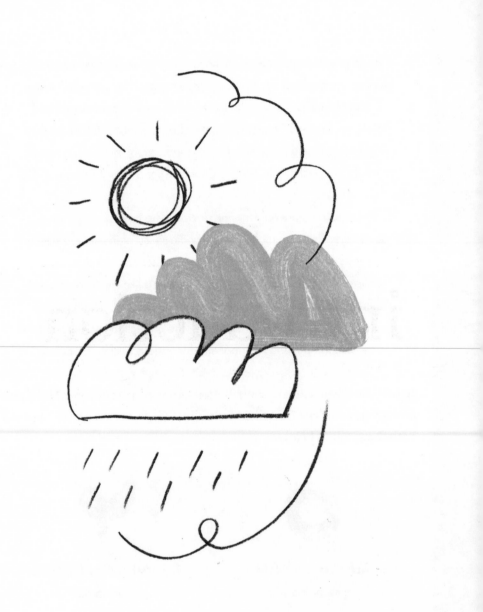

introduction

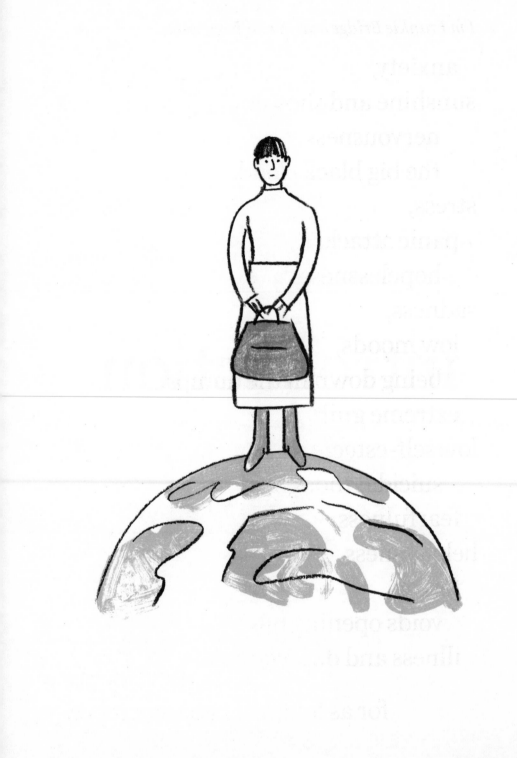

I'm Frankie Bridge and I've suffered with:

anxiety,
sunshine and showers,
nervousness,
the big black cloud,
stress,
panic attacks,
hopelessness,
sadness,
low moods,
being down in the dumps,
extreme guilt,
low self-esteem,
suicidal thoughts,
fearfulness,
helplessness,
terror,
voids opening up,
illness and depression...

for as long as I can remember.

I lived with it
in silence.
I've tried to
conquer it
alone.

Until, eventually, it led to me having a nervous breakdown and being hospitalized at the age of 23. It took me hitting hard, sharp rock bottom, at what was supposed to be the happiest time of my life, for me to truly recognize how ill I had become, and always had been. It took me reaching what could have been my breaking point to begin to take time to help myself and to really get to grips with, and understand, my illness. It's something that I still deal with on a daily basis, and I now know that I will continue to do so for the rest of my life – although I have managed to achieve the things, both professionally and personally, that I have always dreamed of, regardless of the hand my illness has dealt me. My life is not a path I would have chosen, nor would I wish it on anyone else, but I keep on going and I try to live it in the best way I can.

For me, learning about my illness gave me real strength and some much-needed understanding in a confusing, often secretive world. Instead of feeling alone and crazy, I began to realize that so many of us are going through the same thing, but each of us in our own unique way. Getting to know and understand my illness took away my fear of being out of control. *I want you to feel the same.*

In opening up in this book, I want to show you that you are *not alone*, and that we are *all in it together*. Depression, anxiety, panic and deep sadness is an illness just like any other. I want you to know that, while today you may feel like you can't go on and everything is pointless, in an hour, tomorrow, next week, a month from now, you will be able to pick yourself up and things will seem clearer.

With mental health, no one size fits all. It's hard to explain what suffering is like, especially if the person you need to understand you the most has never experienced it themselves. My psychologist once said to me that trying to understand depression by remembering your own sadness is like trying to understand the sensation of drowning by taking a shower. And she's right, but I want to open up the conversation, so we are all better equipped to understand what other people are going through.

It's about breaking down the stigma. Not everything I say will apply to you or those you know because this is my personal journey, but the bare bones of it are the same for us all.

- **We feel helpless**, like nothing we do ever works out and that no one can save us from the deep, dark hole we have got ourselves into.

- **We feel hopeless**, like life will always be this way, so what is the point of trying?

- **We have no interest in anything** that we used to enjoy.

- **We feel that we are useless, a waste of a person**, someone who we and everyone else would be better off without.

- **We suffer from extreme tiredness and lethargy**, so that no matter how much sleep we have, it's never enough. Or we experience the opposite: that no matter how tired we are, we can't sleep.

- **We have an extreme amount of guilt** about everything and anything in our life. Even about the fact that we can't get joy out of the same things that everyone else can.

If any of these symptoms apply to you, or you think this is how someone you know might be feeling, then this is the book for you. Or, if you recognize these traits in people you know, this book will hopefully show you a little bit of how they experience the world. Information is power.

My anxiety controlled me for such a long time because I just didn't understand it. I spent a lot of my childhood trying to dismiss my feelings and anxious, negative thoughts, pushing them to the side, pushing them further and further away, repressing them to the point where I kept silent, adopting – and even becoming – the persona I thought people wanted me to be. I am not sure how I managed to function as a 'normal' human being with such a conflict going on inside my head. So many inner conversations and thoughts, while keeping up a performance all the time.

It honestly wasn't until I had my breakdown that I really got the opportunity to learn what had actually been happening inside my head and to fully understand that it was an illness. That's the problem with having a mental illness; it makes it so hard for you to distinguish between what's real and what's your illness speaking. The mind is a powerful thing, yet we don't listen to it and try to control it. It's amazing that the world is only just starting to realize that understanding what is going on inside is something that needs to be taken really seriously.

Is it because it's so hard to explain?
So hard to understand if you've never felt it?
Because you can't see it?

Physical pain is something we have all experienced at some point in our lives – a headache, nausea, stomach ache – and we all accept this is a real form of pain. We believe and can sympathize with the person who is suffering and, generally, we know how to help them even if they don't ask. If someone has a broken leg and says they're in pain, no one doubts it because they can literally see the cast that shows that the leg has been broken and that your body needs time to heal. The problem with mental illness is that no one can see it.

Mental illness is invisible.

It is invisible. And when you're young, you don't know what it is, so you learn to keep it hidden. You try harder to be better and please more and more people in the hope they will never uncover the 'wrongness', the 'not normal' that exists inside you.

The truth is that I was always an insecure child and girl, and I am still an adult who overthinks situations, who tries her best to please the people around her, but a lot of the thoughts I had early on were directly caused by my illness; my depression and anxiety fuelled my early fears and insecurities. It was my illness, not me, that was convincing me that every bad thought I had about myself was true.

We badly need people like Frankie to help us destigmatize mental illness and to show that people who suffer from it are nevertheless hardworking and highly successful. In choosing to go public with this book, Frankie is making a brave step on both a personal and professional level.

The World Health Organization estimates that there may be over 300 million sufferers from depression in the world today and it is increasingly becoming one of the leading causes of disability worldwide.

Around one in three adults will develop a mental disorder at some point in their life. The three most common conditions are anxiety (12 per cent), depression (9 per cent) and substance-use disorders (10.7 per cent). If we add in other common conditions such as bipolar disorder, schizophrenia, Obsessive Compulsive Disorder (OCD) and dementia, we begin to see that even those who enjoy perfect mental health are usually directly related to someone with a mental illness.

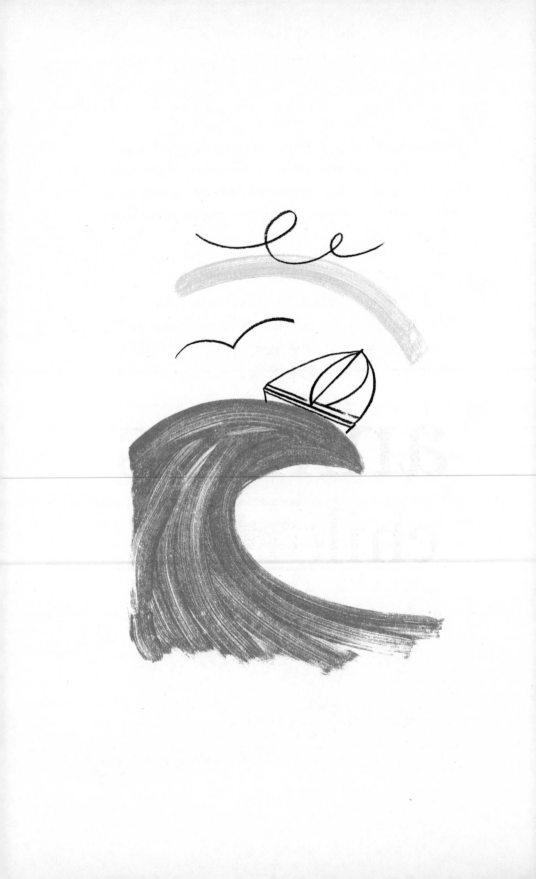

CHAPTER ONE

an
anxious
childhood

AN ANXIOUS CHILDHOOD

Anxiety is usually the state of being afraid when there is nothing to be afraid of.

Why is it that age is how we decide when a person officially becomes an adult? I ask because I can't remember ever feeling like I was a child, or behaving how I would generally imagine a child would behave. The things I did and the life I led, up until I was 12, appeared at a surface level to be typical of a normal childhood, but I don't think my mind and the way I thought about the world were ever how 'normal' children think and feel about their surroundings.

As far back as my mind can stretch, all I remember is that I spent most of my time dreaming up all the bad scenarios that could happen to me, or those around me. When I wasn't conjuring up new disasters, I was worrying about when and how they would take place. Have you ever been terrified watching a horror movie? I feel that sums up the way my brain thinks the world works. Danger at every turn. If my family were planning on going on holiday in the summer, I'd spend the months leading up to it worrying that our plane was going to crash. My imagination, or capacity to see danger in the happy parts of life, knew no limits and if I learned of anything bad happening in the world around me, I would instantly think that it would happen to me next. I became obsessed with spotting the 'danger' around me and began to convince myself that it would take place at any time, which led to me being in a constant state of hyper-alertness. Looking back, I realize I had, from a very young age, managed to master the art of turning something that most people loved and looked forward to into a living nightmare.

Don't get me wrong, I still view my childhood as a happy one. I laughed, I played, I had close relationships with my parents and sister, grandparents and friends. We had a comfortable life and never wanted for anything. However, there was always a battle going on in my mind. I suppose I was a bit like a swan, calm on the surface but paddling like mad underneath, just trying to keep my head above water. As a child, the bonus was that I just had to do what my parents said. I couldn't let the anxiety completely debilitate me. I wasn't making decisions for myself, so I had to just get on with it. If we were going on holiday, I just had to get on that flight with my family.

Death and dying seem to have been deeply rooted in my fears since childhood and I think that fear has always controlled a lot of my thinking. I don't actually know how and when I first learned about death, but it seems I knew very early on that it was our inevitable future and the finality and total unknowability of it terrified me. I do remember going on a school trip to the Imperial War Museum in London. There was a section where you could watch videos and one still replays very clearly in my mind. It was a film of all the dead, naked, emaciated bodies from the concentration camps. They were just being pushed and piled into a massive hole in the ground. Even though I knew this was an extreme circumstance, it frightened me that one minute you're here, a living, breathing human being, and the next you're just a body, skin and bones. Our mortality was completely out of our hands. If that was what happened to us in the end, then I couldn't see the point in life at all.

There were other, physical, signs that I wasn't well from a young age, too. For as long as I can remember, I had stomach aches. It became a bit of a family joke that I basically lived on Pepto-Bismol medicine, but the truth was that if I went without it, I panicked. I was terrified that I might suddenly need the toilet and there would be nowhere for me to go. My mum and I went backwards and forwards to the GP, trying to figure out what was causing my stomach aches, but we never got to the bottom of why they were happening, or what triggered them. I've lost count of the number of blood tests I had, which was another nightmare in itself as I absolutely hated needles. Often, they would have to find extra nurses to hold my arms down during these appointments.

Well-meaning efforts to get the bottom of what was wrong with Frankie became totally counter-productive and the medical tests that were intended to help became part of the problem.

Anxiety sufferers are often over-investigated by their doctors. The succession of doctors and negative tests can have the unfortunate effect of either putting the patient off seeing doctors or, even worse, encouraging them to develop hypochondriacal beliefs – 'What if they've missed something...?' Hypochondriasis is one of a number of medical conditions that doctors can actually cause, or worsen. Among the cures for it is to stop consulting doctors.

After years of stomach aches, my symptoms progressed and worsened. The stomach aches became more frequent and I started having problems with my breathing. I would be fine throughout the day, then the minute I lay down to sleep, my chest would get so incredibly tight that it became harder and harder to pull in any air. No matter how hard I tried, I just couldn't get the deep, full breath I needed. For quite a long time, I struggled in silence with my breathing as I didn't want anyone to know what was going on. Although I was afraid, I felt totally unable to explain this new sensation taking over my body. However, one night I was staying over at my aunt and uncle's house and I kept getting out of bed as the feeling of not being able to breathe had become so uncomfortable and frightening that I couldn't lie still. Eventually I made enough noise to wake my aunt. I remember she looked at me and must have seen that my lips had turned slightly blue, and I recall feeling as though, in that moment, she understood. She took me downstairs, made me a cup of tea and we just chatted until she felt I had evened out. I asked her to keep it between us, so that my parents wouldn't worry. After this, and although the situation continued to scare me, for some reason I still kept it to myself. I did this because I knew, deep down, that something that was deeply rooted inside me was causing it, but I didn't have the words to articulate it, or know what would help the situation, or if anyone would really understand if I said it out loud.

I kept it to myself because I knew, deep down, that something that was deeply rooted inside me was causing it.

And so my breathing issues got worse and worse and the episodes were no longer confined to night-time; they started to happen throughout the day, too. Eventually, I had to tell my parents. I can't remember the conversation, but I know I had just reached the point where I didn't feel like I could hide it any more. I was scared and felt out of control of my own body. So off we went to the doctor's for more rounds of tests. With no explanation, other than diagnosing me as 'a worrier', the doctor gave me an inhaler and sent me and my parents on our way.

The 'worrier' word was used as a way to describe me and my ailments for a long time. It was such a simple word, such a simple way to explain who I was and the cause of my illness, but now I think it was too simplistic to adequately, or accurately, describe what was going on with me. Sitting here writing, I do wonder whether things would have turned out differently for me if mental health had been spoken about back then as it is today. Perhaps I might have been diagnosed with being more than just a worrier? Would my anxiety and panicked states have raised more alarm bells with doctors, and would they have been able to join the dots together more effectively?

Another constant worry that began to fill my thoughts around this time was that no one liked me and that I was a bad person. (Something that has stuck with me and I still battle with today.) Which was ironic as I had always been pretty well liked at school. My solution to my worry that everyone would find out that I truly was a bad person was to try to keep too many people happy at one time – a strategy that inevitably led to letting people down. I think the truth was that, inside, I never felt good enough, or normal enough, and going along with what I thought people wanted was my way of hiding this horrible feeling. I told myself that if I acted the way everyone else wanted me to act, then perhaps they'd never know that I wasn't quite like them and didn't actually belong to the happy world all around me.

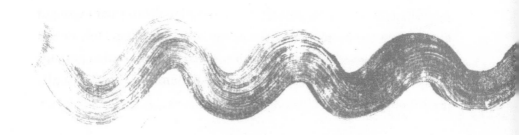

Frankie has grown up always feeling 'less than', or that she is in some way broken inside. Because she is intelligent and perceptive enough to realize that other people simply don't feel that way, her sense of isolation is further increased.

I grew up in Upminster, Essex. Right at the end of the District Line. My parents had moved there from East London a few years before having my sister Tor and me, and it was a really lovely place for us to grow up. It didn't take long to get into London from there, and we could walk to school and into our local town when we needed. We were also never far away from our grandparents and the rest of our family.

I started going to a local dance school when I was three. It was in a local village hall in Cranham. Nothing fancy, but I loved it. A few of my friends went to the same class and we did big shows at the end of every year. My sister Tor came too. We were always really close, considering she is nearly four years older than me. She always let me be included in everything she did with her friends, and she looked after me. Although quite similar in some ways, we're also quite different in so many others.

Especially when it comes to performing and dancing: for her, the dance school was a place to have fun and socialize with her friends. But for me, it was all about the dancing. I took it seriously.

When I was nine, the teacher told my parents she thought they should consider sending me to a stage school. They asked me if it was something I'd like to do. I said yes and we agreed I would audition for the school local to us and if I enjoyed it, I would audition for a bigger, London-based one and go full-time. I got in and loved every minute of it. It was seven hours every Sunday and I auditioned for various parts in the West End and commercials. I often reached the finals but never got the part. I was generally quite resilient to the industry rejection, as I knew and had been told by my parents and teachers that it was just a part of the world I wanted to get into and so I had to get used to it.

My big break came three years later. I'd just had a rejection for the part of Annie in the West End and this time it had hit me hard. It was a part I really wanted, and I remember sobbing in bed, with my mum cuddling me. A few weeks later, I spotted on CBeebies that S Club 7 were holding open auditions for the chance to perform with them at Wembley Arena. Rochelle Humes – or Rochelle Wiseman, as she was back then – was a really good friend of mine. Little did we know that so much of our future would be intertwined: we would end up being in not one, but two successful pop groups together.

Rochelle and I were at the same stage school at the time and we managed to convince our mums to take us along to the auditions. After a few weeks of callbacks, we got in! And it turned out that we were not only going to go on tour with S Club 7, but also becoming part of an actual pop group! We couldn't believe it. I remember realizing that if I had got that part in *Annie*, then I would never have auditioned for S Club Juniors and I was amazed at how the world worked, how sometimes bad luck could allow for good luck to follow. I totally believed it was fate and was meant to be. I had no idea how much my life was about to change.

I had no idea how much my life was about to change.

A few days later, we went to a family party. I can remember all the adults discussing their general worry that I might get into drugs or end up with an eating disorder, which were the main things child stars had been reported to have dealt with at that time. My dad said that the minute he saw me not eating, he'd pull me out. It must have been such a tough decision for them – they either had to allow me to leave school and pretty much hand me over to someone who would thrust me out into the spotlight, or say no and run the risk of me resenting them for the rest of their lives. At the time, I didn't appreciate how tough this must have been for them, but now I'm a parent myself, I don't think it's a choice I would like to face. It must have caused them so much worry and stress.

Looking back now, I feel truly sorry for my younger self. I was going through a lot but was also hiding a lot about myself from the world around me. I was worried all the time and had this burning sensitivity to the dangers of everyday life, not just for me but for my family and friends too. Although I did try and share some of my worries with the people I was closest to, it became a bit of a joke in the end, mainly because I never really shared how deeply these thoughts were buried within me and I allowed people to think they were just surface concerns. People probably just thought they were fleeting moments of anxiety from a kid with a very vivid imagination. On the outside, I just looked like I had developed some peculiar little habits. For quite a long time, I insisted on sleeping inside my duvet cover, as close to the wall as possible, just in case a bomb fell or someone broke into the house. I never actually told anyone the reason why I had taken to behaving in these self-protective ways because, at the time, it made complete sense to me. I didn't feel I needed to explain myself to anybody.

Obsessional thoughts are common in childhood, but most children can usually forget all about them quite quickly. In Frankie's mind, everyday fears and anxieties that others brush off easily had a tendency to grow roots and not to shift at all.

People often ask me why, considering the way I am, I decided to go into the entertainment industry, but actually, I feel as though a lot of people in this business are wired like me. Maybe it's the desire for acceptance, a way of fulfilling that constant need to make other people happy? Maybe it was the thought of seeing the smiles on people's faces during a performance or at a meet and greet, or hearing the applause at the end of a show, that drove me towards my career, in the hope that one day I would finally feel accepted? Being on stage felt like I was playing a character, I wasn't really me when I was performing. It was really freeing to think solely about the songs and the dance moves. I didn't have time to think about any of my worries. It was my form of escape.

Although my job probably didn't help my illness, the anxiety was ingrained in me already and I believe that I would have reached breaking point at some point in my life regardless of my early childhood success. It just would have been something else that tipped me over the edge. I feel as though my time in S Club Juniors was probably when I was at my healthiest, mentally. We were so well looked after, I was surrounded by an amazing team of adults on a daily basis and I was doing what I loved every day. I also feel a big part of my contentment was the absence of social media. I had no idea what people thought of me or my band; if they liked our songs, me, or the way I looked. There were no online articles to pull me up on every misplaced hair, dodgy vocal or bad life decision and I never really had any idea of the scale of our success at that time. I was left alone in my own happy bubble.

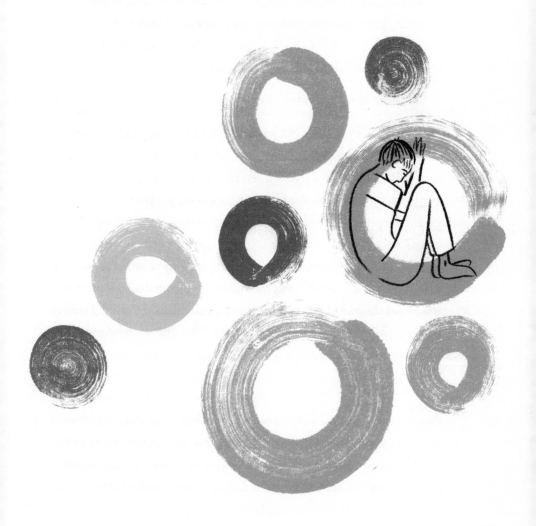

WORRIERS

Anxiety disorders can affect around 30 per cent of children under the age of 18 at some point in their lives. Common symptoms of Generalized Anxiety Disorder (or GAD, as it is known for short) in children and adolescents are:

- Worrying about things before they happen – what if? When?

- Worrying about friends, family safety, school or activities

- Having a phobia about death

- Frequent stomach aches, headaches or other physical symptoms

- Sleep disturbance

- Excessive worry about sleeping away from home

- Clingy behaviour with family members

Sometimes a child (or adult) can be characterized as a 'worrier', but it's helpful to know the signs to look out for that may indicate a bigger problem. When worrying becomes extreme, there is a tendency to catastrophize and over-analyse risks (even where there are none). This can be debilitating, as excessive concerns of abandonment or danger can take over logical thought.

People with Generalized Anxiety Disorder tend to catastrophize outcomes, overestimating the danger and underestimating their ability to cope. Research suggests that worriers need to be completely sure that they are making the right decision and are reluctant to accept uncertainty, which means they will often delay making a decision about solving the issues and go into their default mechanism of thinking about all the things that can go wrong. They adopt 'safety behaviours', trying to predict problems, avoiding risky situations and looking for reassurance from others.

Once a 'worrier' starts overthinking an issue in this way, and dwelling on what they think could (or did) go wrong, they can become paralysed and unable to get on with their life.

Problem-solving is the antidote to most worries, but while worriers are relatively good at identifying problems, they are incredibly bad at solving them. Indecision tends to paralyse worriers and they end up going over and over the bad consequences of certain life events, a process psychologists call 'ruminating'.

Often it's a matter of wanting to control uncontrollable events, rather than learning to accept and reframe them.

Inevitable life events such as death and the illness of loved ones are a common concern of worriers, who want to control the future. Psychology has developed the idea of Acceptance and this would be a good area to apply it to. We can't do anything about death, but we can change how we feel about it by encouraging ourselves to accept it peacefully and not be afraid of its inevitability. This is not a religious concept, but a reframing of the idea of threat.

sunshine and showers

My nan – Nanny Honey Bunny, as we called her – was a major part of my life when I was growing up. She and my grandad Ron, who were my mum's parents, often helped out with childcare. They would pick us up from school and we'd often go and stay at their house when my parents were out at work. We loved them. They were everything grandparents should be – caring, loving and funny, turning everything into a song – and we loved to be in their company. I remember my nan would stand me on the side of the sofa and tell me to stop growing, which always made me laugh. In fact, she'd often stroke my head until I fell asleep (something that I now make my husband Wayne do to me, much to his dismay, but it always chills me out and sends me to sleep) and they always went above and beyond to make sure that I felt very secure and loved. Although I wasn't aware of it at the time, I think she was the first person to figure me out, almost as though she knew who I was even before I did. She knew I needed that extra level of care.

Her name for me was 'Sunshine and Showers' and it wasn't until just before she passed away about 15 years later that I realized she had managed to sum me up perfectly from the start. Perhaps she had always known that I wasn't like the other children and this was her way of expressing it to me.

The nickname 'Sunshine and Showers' is playful and reassuring – we all know that showers don't last long, and that the sun will soon be out again. Sadly, the reality for Frankie was that the showers were prolonged and heavy, and sooner or later a full-blown storm was to come.

Frankie is a naturally sunny personality. When she is sad, she is slow to blame others and quick to criticize herself.

It feels like my life has always been in a state of 'Sunshine and Showers'. My mood is either up or down, I'm loud and energetic or I'm quiet and want to be alone, I either *love* you or I *hate* you. There's not much of a grey area with me, I am made up of extremes. Nan's phrase has defined me and my life so much that I have it tattooed across my back. Sadly, by the time I got to show her, her dementia had advanced too far, but that was what she'd always called me and 'sunshine and showers' will always be one of the best ways of explaining my story to you: a life of ups and downs.

Sunlight and stormy clouds. Happiness and sadness.

OPEN NOTES

Childhood depression affects around 1 per cent of pre-pubertal children and up to 3 per cent of adolescents. It is at least twice as common in girls as in boys. The diagnosis is based on feeling, or appearing, depressed, sad, tearful or irritable and:

- Not enjoying things as much as before

- Spending less time with friends or in school activities

- Changes in appetite and/or weight

- Sleeping more, or less, than usual

- Feeling tired or having less energy

- Feeling like everything is their fault or they're not good at anything

- Having more trouble concentrating

- Caring less about school, or not doing as well at school

- Having thoughts about suicide or wanting to die

Childhood depression is an under-diagnosed condition as medical professionals are usually slow to notice it, and even when we do observe the symptoms, we tend to put them down to developmental, friendship or relationships issues, or problems at school. However, only around 60 per cent of children fully recover within a year from the onset of the illness and in a good many cases, it is the first warning sign of a recurring, and sometimes lifelong, condition that has to be managed, rather than something that will simply go away as they grow up.

Depression and anxiety are conditions that have a dramatic effect on our thoughts and the way we look at things. If we develop the illness in childhood, before our personality has begun to form, the depressed thinking will have an enormous impact on the way we will always look at the world. We may see it as a threatening and frightening place. In such a case, the illness will affect not just our day-to-day functioning, it will begin to change who and what we are. We may be left guessing what others think and feel compelled to pretend to be like them in order to fit in.

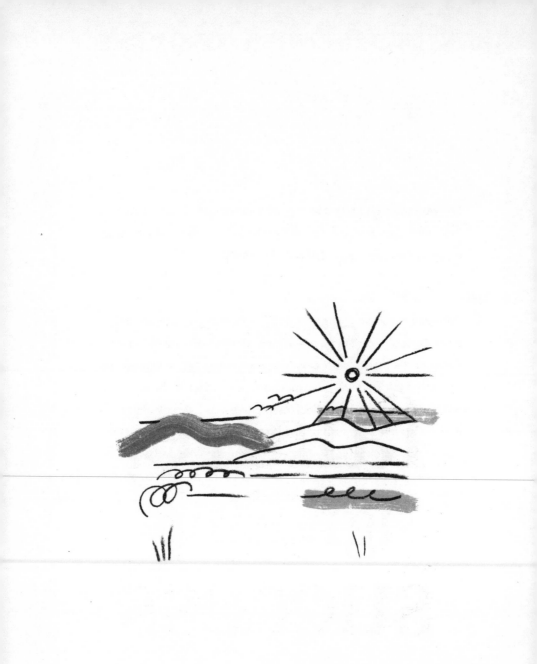

seeing failure, ignoring success

CHAPTER TWO

SEEING FAILURE, IGNORING SUCCESS

One of my biggest 'ups' was joining The Saturdays in 2007. We were put together by a record label, Universal – the same people that had signed S Club Juniors. They rang me while I was on holiday in Zante with a friend, trying to be a 'normal' teenager. They asked if I could come in to see them when I was back, as they were putting together a new girl band and thought I would be perfect for it. I was anxious about being in another group situation, but I was so unclear about what my future was going to hold that I felt as though I was in no position to say no.

When I got back home, I went to see the people at the record label. Their idea sounded great, and it also felt good to be back working with a lot of the same people as before. Two of my friends had travelled into London with me and when I came out of the meeting, I just remember saying, 'I think I'm in a girlband'. It was so surreal. A few weeks later, me and about six other girls were being put through our paces, singing and dancing together. Seeing how we all blended together and who worked with who. At that age, althoughI would get nervous in audition situations, I don't ever remember doubting my abilties as a performer. Eventually, they chose the four other girls that I would go on to spend a lot of time with. I don't think at the time I really took in how lucky I was to be back on this journey again. My friends were all about to go off to uni or work and here I was about to start yet another pop career. It was exciting, but you're always aware in the back of your mind that it might not be successful, it may fail.

After all the excitement, I think we ended up waiting near on a year to actually start doing any work together. But once we started, we took every gig going, travelling up and down the country to perform in nightclubs, universities – wherever would have us – and rehearsing in between. We never turned anything down because, the way we saw it, every gig was a chance to be seen and heard by someone new and could take us a step closer to where we wanted and needed to be. We absolutely loved it and had a lot of fun, but it was relentlessly hard work and I found it mentally and physically exhausting and draining.

After a few years of trying to keep up with this unstoppable pace, I began to find myself unable to commit to a performance. The thing that I had always loved to do, and had spent my whole life working for, suddenly started to seem impossible. The thing that would usually be my form of release from all the thoughts in my head, the place where I could become a different person, had now become the thing that filled me with dread. I would give everything I had to my vocals and dance routines, not forgetting the all-important, ever constant smile, but my mind was elsewhere, questioning everything, everyone and mostly myself. I began to worry that people thought I didn't look any good. If they thought I sounded as bad as I felt I did. If they believed, as I did, that I didn't deserve to be up on that stage, that I was a fraud. Having previously been in a child band, I had been given a second shot at pop stardom and I knew just how lucky I was, but I also knew just how quickly the whole thing could fail and collapse around me. I never allowed myself just to live in the moment, to soak it all up. It became a battleground between me, my anxieties and I.

○

At this stage in Frankie's life, the first signs of Negative Automatic Thoughts (NATs) are creeping in. NATs cause sufferers to ignore positive or neutral information and instead focus on negative events and comments. Examples of NATs are:

- OVER-GENERALIZING – if one thing goes wrong, everything will go wrong
- PERSONALIZING – interpreting negative events as confirmation of worthlessness
- CATASTROPHIZING – always imagining the worst case scenario
- MIND READING – assuming people know what we think and how we are feeling

In depression and anxiety, NATs may appear reasonable, but in fact, the more we listen to and believe these thoughts, the worse we feel. For Frankie, ordinary performance anxiety has become something much worse and she is now having difficulty in believing that she has any talent at all. She also catastrophizes, imagining something bad happening during the performance – forgetting her lines, forgetting the choreography, having a panic attack – that would result in her being publicly humiliated and people thinking she has gone mad.

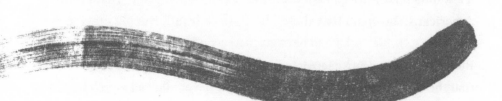

Things came to a head at a rehearsal. We were in our usual studios in London and had an upcoming show in a nightclub. We'd been discussing how tired and mentally drained we all felt and realized that there was no way we'd be able to do the show the fans deserved and that if we didn't make a stand to stop it now, we never would be able to. So we made the decision to speak to our manager and asked her to cancel the show. She told us that the only way we could pull out without any backlash was to get letters from our GPs to say that we physically couldn't do it. We would be in breach of our contracts otherwise and people were expecting to see us perform. We had to have a valid reason not to do the show, substantiated by medical professionals.

As soon as I got into the GP's room, I burst into tears. I sobbed uncontrollably.

We all booked our appointments to see a doctor. I was expecting to simply explain how unbelievably mentally and physically exhausted I felt and be told to take a day off. But as soon as I got into the GP's room, I burst into tears. I sobbed uncontrollably. I could hardly get my words out. It was as though all the feelings I'd spent my whole life suppressing were rising up and bubbling over. I couldn't stop them. Sitting in that room, I felt at my most helpless and very exposed and vulnerable. The GP listened and told me that he thought I was suffering from more than just exhaustion and that he felt I should go and see a counsellor. I couldn't compute it. I was just overtired and needed to take a few days off. Please could it just be that simple. Only crazy people, or Americans, saw therapists and I was neither of those, so why would I?

But, deep, deep, deep, deep down, at the very back of my mind, I knew that the GP was right. I became more aware of my behaviour. Although

What was the
matter with
me?
This couldn't
be happening.

I kept on holding everything together when I was at work, I noticed that, when I came home, I was incapable of eating dinner and I couldn't make conversation. I just went straight to bed and cried myself to sleep.

After a few weeks, my boyfriend at the time and I sat down and talked about what was going on with me. We agreed that the way I was feeling couldn't be right. When the doctor had said I needed therapy it was easy to dismiss it – he'd only seen me for a matter of minutes after all – but it was scary to know that someone I was so close to had also seen such a negative change in me. I had reached the point where something had to change.

It took a lot out of me, but I knew I couldn't go on the way I had been, so I took the plunge and started seeing a therapist that the GP had recommended. I didn't question his choice because I had absolutely no idea where to find one myself.

The truth is, the decision to see someone made me feel even more of a failure. Counselling just wasn't what 'normal' people did, none of my friends had to do it and it didn't fit with who I was supposed to be. All those years of trying to be the best person I could be – the girl from Essex who had managed to carve out not one, but two, pop careers for herself. The girl who was 'living the dream' was so incredibly unhappy. The life so many were desperate to lead, the life *I* was desperate to lead, just wasn't enough. My constant struggle to be my version of perfect had failed. I felt I had become a typical child star who couldn't cope with the fame and success and I felt embarrassed that I was becoming everything I never thought I would. I was failing at life even when at the top.

As someone struggling with generalized anxiety, Frankie had very low self-confidence and self-worth. As is very common with anxious people, she believed that she had been lucky to have any success and it was nothing to do with hard work.

The trouble is, I'm a perfectionist. On the plus side, this personality trait has helped me succeed because it means that I have never, ever, stopped striving, but it has also been a major contributor to my anxiety. It's the reason for much of my stress and for my overwhelming feelings of failure. It stops me from ever being able to look at my life and feel that I did my best, that I've achieved as much as I could have done. It keeps pushing me on, but it also stops me from ever realizing how far I have come and it stops me putting myself out there to try new things.

This isn't only with regards to my career, it applies to my personal life too. I will always try to give 100 per cent of myself to everything I do, even though I know that it isn't realistic or sustainable. People can tell me until they're blue in the face that I've done a great job, that I'm a good friend/mother/wife/pretty much anything, but I will never believe them because I will always think of the bits I could have done better, or differently; of the failures rather than the successes.

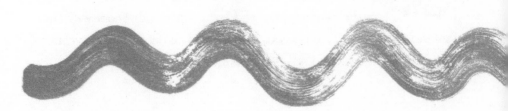

People with low self-esteem hold back from life. Treating it requires us to act differently and to try things even though we might fail. In other words, no matter how inadequate a person we feel we might be, we have to act as though we have a liking and respect for ourselves.

People with depression are often ashamed of their psychological distress and society makes it taboo to admit it openly. Shame makes us think of ourselves as subordinate in some way where people with depression feel judged by society in a negative way so much so that they can feel ostracized and inferior.

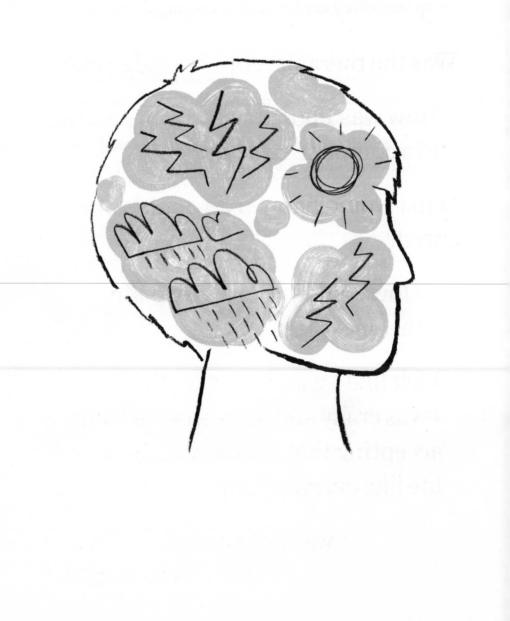

my first therapy session

I was incredibly nervous going into my first session.

Was the therapist going to judge me?

How was I possibly going to open up
to a complete stranger?

What would happen if I couldn't be
cured?

How could I begin to explain
the unexplainable?

I felt like I was accepting that
I was crazy and admitting defeat;
accepting that I couldn't cope with
life like everyone else.

I was not normal.

I was not OK.

Therapy wasn't what I had expected; there wasn't a loud ticking clock on the wall, or a chaise longue in front of a window for me to lie on – although the therapist did ask, 'And how did that make you feel?' Mostly, it was a normal conversation, albeit with someone you were paying and didn't know at all! It felt incredibly surreal at first, to go and sit in a room with a stranger and reveal my deepest and darkest thoughts – thoughts I'd barely managed confess to myself, let alone tell those closest to me – but I got used to it and the more I overcame my fears and opened up, the more benefits I felt from just speaking to someone out loud.

O

When people arrive in therapy, they are often scared, confused and ashamed. Many are also under the misconception that they are the only ones who have ever felt such pain, fear and sense of loss. However, the symptoms and feelings they describe are often familiar to me, because I have heard their stories before, many times. People with OCD hide behaviour for weeks before admitting to it, partly because they are not ready to give it up but mainly because of shame. Anxious people tell me that they must be wasting my time, because their problems are silly and there are others who are really unwell. I've heard this from so many people, Frankie being one of them.

I went every week for quite a long time, making sure work knew I needed to make time for it in my hectic schedule, but after a few months I realized that, while it was good to talk, I still wasn't getting back to 'normal'. I was talking but not getting better. At this point, I had no idea that people tried out different therapists before finding the right match. I just assumed that these things take time and that I was expecting too much too soon, so I persevered, rather than asking myself whether this therapist was the right person for me to speak to.

Seeking out psychotherapy is something of a minefield in the UK because it is not a regulated industry. I would advise against searching for a therapist on the internet, but instead get a recommendation from a doctor, hospital or insurance company that has had regular contact with the practitioner and is in a position to get feedback about their work.

There had been an option to try medication from the get-go, but at the time it felt like too drastic a step to take without therapy first. I felt I had to try to get better by myself, after all this was just a *feeling*, I wasn't actually ill, so why would I go on medication? And I believed, and hoped, that I'd be back to normal after a few weeks of therapy. I think maybe the therapist saw that I needed more from the start, but I was scared. I didn't like the idea of taking a pill that could change my mood – what if I became numb, vacant and quiet? Hardly useful characteristics for someone who entertains the public for a living! I didn't know anyone who took antidepressants, and it seemed as if everyone I spoke to had such an aversion to them, that no one really accepted depression as an actual illness, or they were something you should only take for a short period of time and under no circumstances stay on for the rest of your life. And if I'm being honest, I think I felt that if I really needed the medication, then I must have failed again because I had failed to get better on my own. It seemed that my health was just another task that I had to be perfect at. And needed to overcome without help.

But eventually I had had enough of feeling so low. I felt as though I just couldn't cope with it any more, so I gave in and admitted that therapy just wasn't enough. I wanted to try the medication as well. It was such a relief to finally give in, it felt like I was taking a big helpful step forward.

Little did I know that this would be the start of an even longer journey. Because it turns out that just as one particular psychologist or type of therapy is not right for everyone, one medicine doesn't fit all either.

The first thing I tried was Prozac. That's what pretty much everyone seems to start on at the beginning and it worked at first, but in my case, it certainly didn't do the job.

At some point I gave up. Nothing seemed to be making any difference, so I took myself off the Prozac, stopped seeing my therapist and decided to go it alone.

Antidepressant medication usually takes 10–14 days to have much of an effect on mood, and the dose often has to be adjusted upwards or downwards every week or two in order to balance benefits against any side effects. It can be many weeks before the medication reaches full effect, though it is usually obvious within two weeks if a particular dose is actually helping. Around one-third of people treated with antidepressants have a useful response but do not enter full remission.

Because we know that psychotherapy, like medication, seldom works within a day or two of beginning, we are wary of any dramatic improvement after the first tablet or initial session. This is usually a false dawn brought about by the relief of meeting someone who seems to understand and to want to help. We would usually regard this as a 'flight into health' in which the patient is wishfully thinking their problems away, or a 'placebo response', in which the patient is responding to the doctor, not the medication.

I thought,
well,
I've got this far
without pills
or therapy
after all.
This turned out
to be a very bad
decision.

panic

Alongside the diagnosis of depression, there had been another unwelcome addition to my life: panic attacks. These attacks would seemingly come out of nowhere but they tended to follow one of my uncontrollable crying sessions. My chest would start to feel heavy and tight and I would feel as if I couldn't catch a breath, a breath deep enough to fill my lungs and keep me breathing, keep me living. It was so frightening that I'd panic that I couldn't breathe at all, which made matters ten times worse. The sensation would make me feel so unbelievably helpless, as though I had absolutely no control over my mind or body. *It was all-consuming and utterly terrifying.*

But still I kept it hidden. It was my terrible secret and not something I would share with my friends and family. How could *anyone* possibly understand what was going on if I didn't understand myself? And anyway, I had no idea what they were, what they were called or what would bring them on, so how could I even begin to explain them to anyone else? Not being in control, never knowing when one of these episodes would strike, left me in a constant state of fear.

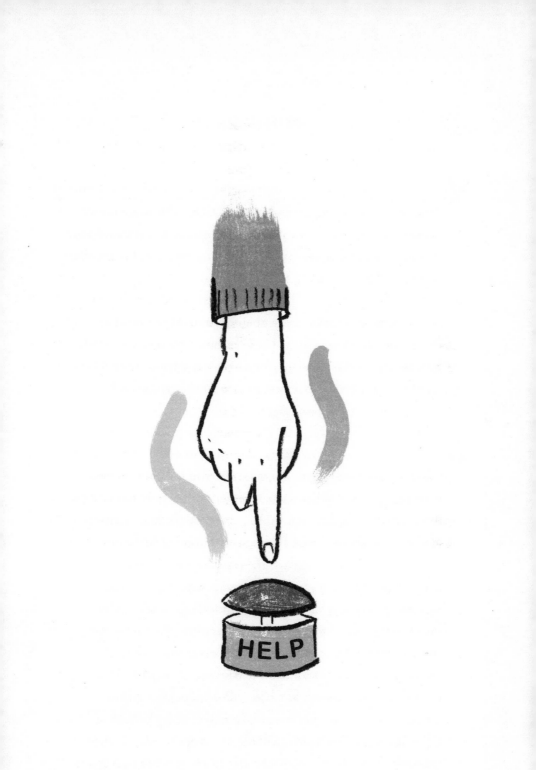

OPEN NOTES

Panic attacks are utterly terrifying. It is like being hit by a mental tsunami: all ability to think rationally is swept away and the sufferer is forced to stop whatever they are doing in order to try to control the feelings in their mind and body.

They often believe that they are about to pass out, or even die. There is an immediate urge to flee from the situation, to get away from other people and out into the fresh air and quiet. A good many sufferers will call an ambulance, so sure are they that something is terribly, terribly wrong with them.

Our body and brain have developed effective systems to respond to physical danger. When we see a threat, the acute stress response kicks in and our bodies experience a chain of reactions, enabling us to fight or flee the danger, through the release of the hormones adrenaline and noradrenaline. The first thing that happens is that the heart starts to beat very fast, pumping more blood into our muscles and causing our blood vessels to dilate – which is why we start to feel so hot. We start to breathe faster, our throats become dry and our chest feels tight, triggering fear because evolution has taught us to protect our heart and lungs. We might also feel butterflies in our stomach as blood is diverted away from the digestive system – we don't need to be eating or drinking while we're fighting or fleeing from danger! It is a perfect alarm system. However, human beings now react not only to real threats, but also to imagined threats, which evolution didn't really design it for. We can imagine humiliation, we can worry about future events, we can visualize the plane crashing or the train becoming stuck in a tunnel. And sure enough our dutiful brain and body go into alarm mode.

Panic attacks are not 'all in the mind'. They are accompanied by powerful physical sensations because the mind and body are connected – just remember a time when you have been on a roller coaster or watched a scary movie; the fear and excitement probably caused your heart to pound and your breathing to increase because your body released adrenaline. When people experience panic attacks, they often become terrified and feel that they're about to die. This in itself is a terrifying thought, which itself leads to more panic symptoms.

Most people who have the correct form of psychological therapy can go on and have a life free from panic. The most effective form of treatment for panic is Cognitive Behavioural Therapy, which focuses on understanding what is happening in our bodies, but most importantly, the relationship between thoughts and anxiety.

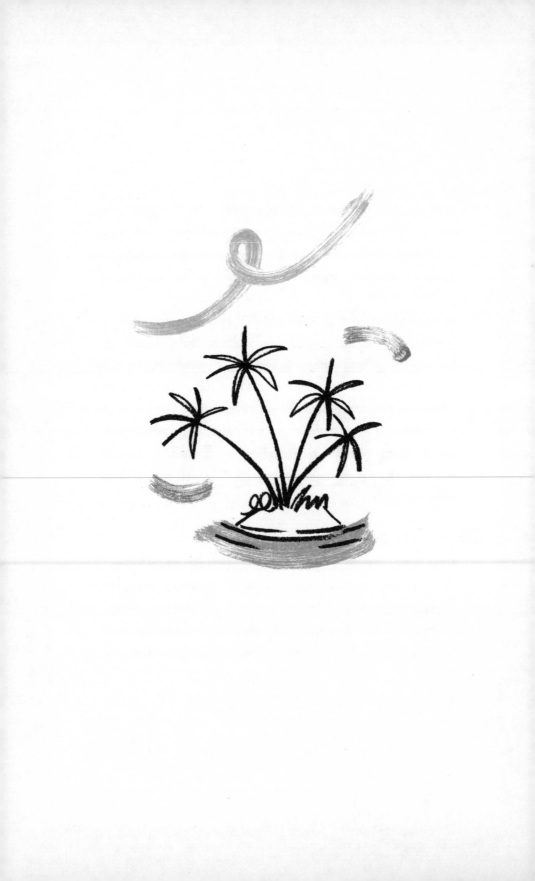

CHAPTER THREE

staying silent

STAYING SILENT

Anxiety, panic and depression were part of my daily life, but still I managed to carry on performing.

The Saturdays were big – our début single had made the Top 10, and after that the hits just kept on coming. I've never been a serious partyer – parties fill me with all sorts of anxieties – and I have a phobia of being sick, so I don't drink much. I don't like the feeling of being out of control. But going out was part of living the pop-star dream, wasn't it? This was how I was meant to live. And we were so well looked after – free drinks, no queuing. Going out became a new norm for me. Perhaps it was another means of escaping from myself.

It was a good distraction too, a way of avoiding things at home. Things weren't going too well in my relationship and it had become a source of real heartbreak for me. My partner was someone I thought I would be with forever. We'd liked each other from afar for years and both believed we were meant to be. I couldn't believe my luck when we finally got together. When your work life is so busy, relationships seem to develop a lot faster than usual, because you have less time to hang out and figure it all out slowly. Having the whole world watching and waiting, documenting every moment, doesn't help either. I moved in with him pretty quickly and his friends and band members became my extended family. It felt so nice to be with someone who understood my life, who knew how busy I was and had experienced the highs and lows of the industry himself. We'd both started out at a similar age, so I felt we just got each other.

However, after a few years things started unravelling – we were both young pop stars, constantly in the spotlight, and it turned out that we were battling some pretty big mental demons too. Looking back now, I realize that I was in such a rush to grow up and live the life I thought a pop star should be living. I thought we needed the big house, the flashy car, the fancy holidays, when none of those things were really what either of us was about, or what we needed to make us happy. We went through some big, hard experiences as a couple, things that even people much older than us wouldn't have been able to deal with. Things we went through silently, separately. We were two people at their weakest, trying to hold each other up, without actually speaking out and telling each other what we were going through individually. The break-up hit us both pretty hard, and it came at a point in our lives when neither of us could really cope with much more. A huge failure that I still carry with me and that has shaped a lot of my life since, in good and bad ways.

My partner and I were two people at their weakest, trying to hold each other up.

It was around this point that the partying stepped up a level. I was on seven days a week of nights out. I was not eating, I was binge drinking and looking for reassurance and confidence in all the wrong guys (a new escape to calm my overthinking mind), and still working every day. I may have looked like I was having a great time, but I was so lost and confused. I had spent so many years picturing what my life was going to look like and now I'd messed it all up. I hated myself and I definitely couldn't imagine anyone else being able to love me ever again. I wasn't worthy of it.

One night my best friend and I were on one of our usual evenings out. All of a sudden I felt overwhelmed with emotions. I took myself off to the toilets and collapsed on the floor of a cubicle. I felt that I had nothing left to give. I felt completely out of control of my own mind and body. I had no idea who I was anymore. I didn't like who I'd become. It was as if my body and mind were no longer mine and my body just took over. I couldn't breathe and my mind was racing, but empty. The sobs just flew out of me, as if every single emotion I had been holding in just couldn't be contained anymore. My friend came and found me. She was shocked, because she had never seen me like this before. She later told me that it was if any tiny shred of confidence I had left had disappeared and I was a shell of myself. It was the first time she realized how fragile I had become. She literally picked me up off the floor and took me home.

Despite this, I continued to work and go on nights out, drowning my sorrows and trying to push those feelings of self-hatred back down. Little did I know that I would soon meet Wayne Bridge – my knight in shining armour. It was pretty soon after my break-up and I had absolutely no intention of meeting someone new, as I was totally broken from my last relationship, but sometimes things happen when you least expect them. We met through a mutual friend on a night out and had a laugh, but nothing more than that. After a few weeks of blowing him off – he was a footballer, so I just assumed he was bad news – I got in touch. After chatting constantly for days and him hinting that he wanted to take me out, I suggested we should go out for dinner. He'd been so lovely and kind, despite my rudeness. We arranged to go to a favourite place we both had in common – a Japanese restaurant called Zuma in London. I turned up 45 minutes late, but he didn't seem to mind, and we had an amazing time, chatting until the restaurant closed.

It was just after Christmas and he headed straight back from London to Manchester that night, as he had training the next day and that was where he was living at the time. A day after that, I drove north to see him and ended up staying until I had to go back to London for work several weeks later. It was quite full on, but you don't get much downtime in our jobs, so we had to take the opportunity on offer to get to know each other properly.

I was totally broken from my last relationship, but sometimes things happen when you least expect them.

One week in, we were spotted together by the press. There were lots of online articles full of snide comments about how quickly we'd got together after my break-up with my previous boyfriend, which played into all my insecurities, but I was happy and it was all so unexpected. He was a footballer, so friends and family wanted to dislike him, but if you ever have the pleasure of meeting Wayne, you'll understand that it's pretty much impossible to find anything to dislike about him. I felt we had a lot in common, in that we'd both worked from a young age and committed most our lives to our careers. We just clicked.

One night during those first months together, we were in a restaurant having a great time, still wrapped up in that honeymoon phase of a new relationship. I suddenly started getting text messages from friends, telling me that they had seen on social media and in the press that my previous boyfriend had had to go into rehab. It was an incredibly hard way to find out such intimate news about the man I had lived with and who I had been with for so long, someone I truly cared about, regardless of the way things had ended. It killed me that he was in such a bad way, so unhappy, and that there was nothing I could do to help. In truth, it hurt almost as much as the news itself – along with the fact that I was getting blamed by all the online keyboard warriors.

Of course, I instantly blamed myself, so the public judgements only made things worse. I hated that I had become someone in his life that no one saw worthy of being told the news. After years of therapy, I now know that unfortunately it was already the way he was heading, but at the time I had absolutely no idea what was going on. Rightly or wrongly, Wayne and I decided to work our way through the entire cocktail menu, which seemed like the only way to deal with it at the time. Just to block it all out. This was a really difficult and sad time in my life. I was embarrassed for Wayne to see something that at the time I believed I had caused. It was an awkward situation for a relatively new relationship: no one likes to talk about their partner's past, let alone have to deal with it in the present. I had been totally open with Wayne beforehand, so he knew all about my previous relationship, which probably helped us to handle it as a couple. The next morning, however, I had my first ever proper hangover. And, of course, nothing had become easier to deal with.

Of course, I instantly blamed myself, so the public judgements only made things worse.

But despite this overwhelming sadness, I also knew that Wayne was just what I needed. So laid-back, funny, not in my industry, kind, thoughtful and someone who could take control and ownership of situations. I didn't have to think with him, I felt looked-after and safe. He is eight years older than me and, although I never noticed the age difference in a negative way, I did feel like he was more mature and that he knew who he was – which was very different to how I felt about myself, as below the surface the struggle was ever present.

Things have never been plain sailing with us, but Wayne and I have both fought for each other. We both came with our own baggage and insecurities from past relationships and it has taken us a long time to break down barriers and figure out what the other needs. For instance, Wayne found it really hard to tell me he loved me for a really long time. He used to say 'I hate you' instead, but we both knew what he really meant, though. I was happy to wait for him to decide in his own time when he was able to actually say 'I love you' because I already knew he did. That's how I knew he was someone special. Things weren't perfect, but they were right, and I knew we could get through it all and, more importantly, I wanted to. I love to be around people who teach me new things and push me to do things I wouldn't normally do because I'm someone who could easily hide and stick to the things I know, but Wayne pushed through those boundaries. We began to build a life together.

But after about a year of being together, my old, dark ways of thinking and feeling started creeping back in. I remember being in the shower in the beautiful house we now shared and I just had this realization that something wasn't right. I was so happy, but I knew I should be happier. I loved this man, I loved my job. But I was sad to my very core. It's so hard to explain unless you've felt this sensation.

How can
   you be so happy,
but at the
     same time
     be so
deeply and
     painfully
        unhappy?

I was so frustrated with myself. What was it going to take for me to feel the happiness I knew I should? But in my usual manner, I ignored the feelings and brushed them to the side. I was ashamed and to be quite honest, I just didn't want to look at them too deeply.

The so called 'love drug' is very powerful. Strong hormones and neurotransmitters like oxytocin and dopamine flood our brains when we fall in love. Most of us have experienced the extreme happiness and optimism that come with a new love relationship, and in Frankie's case, it clearly counteracted her depression for many months. Although we like to pretend that it is not so, the reality is that being in love slowly gives way to loving someone, which is a much more peaceful, enduring and contented feeling. Loving someone gives us strength, but it is not usually enough on its own to fight off a severe depression.

CLINICAL DEPRESSION

One of the worst and most counterproductive symptoms of depression is the feeling of being totally alone. The sense that no one else will understand, or care, how you feel is often the reason why those suffering with it don't speak out. Talking to someone – anyone – is a huge step towards feeling better; it's the way to start dragging yourself out of that deep, dark hole. But when you're in that hole, speaking out feels like the hardest thing in the world.

Depression is a state of mind we are all vulnerable to. No one is sufficiently robust to be immune. Life events, losses and/or childhood trauma can affect our state of mind, which becomes imbalanced. This then impacts on our mood, our thinking and our behaviour.

According to The American Psychiatric Association, a person can be said to suffer from a major depression if during a two-week period, they demonstrate a change from previous functioning and experience either a depressed mood (that is to say, they feel sad or empty) most of the day or nearly every day, or a markedly diminished interest or pleasure in all, or almost all, activities most of the day.

This must be accompanied by at least four of the below:

- Either a change in appetite nearly every day or significant weight loss when not dieting, or weight gain (a change of more than 5 per cent of body weight in a month)

- Insomnia or hypersomnia

- Psychomotor agitation (purposeless movements such as pacing or tapping) or retardation. (This must be observable by others, not merely subjective feelings of restlessness or being slowed down.)

- Fatigue or loss of energy nearly every day
- Feelings of worthlessness, excessive or inappropriate guilt
- Diminished ability to think or concentrate, or indecisiveness
- Recurrent thoughts of death and suicidal ideation, with or without a specific plan.

In a depressed state, we are consumed by thoughts of 'Why bother? Nothing will change. What's the point?' People stop self-care, avoid social situations, stop cleaning their living space – all because of the booming and self-destructive thoughts. They start to magnify the difficulty of tasks and believe that they won't be able to complete them (probably to their high perfectionist levels).

Depressed people feel illogical, irrational and unhelpful shame over faults and failings that almost everyone else has. They crucify themselves mentally because of this.The entirely useless load of guilt and shame acts like a backpack full of rocks in their journey through life. Cognitive Behavioural Therapy aims to help them simply take off the backpack, leave it by the side of the road and walk on unburdened. It really is as simple – and as difficult – as that.

The problem is that those of us who have never had depression tend to try and imagine it by remembering a time when we were very sad. While ordinary human sadness and depression do have some things in common, it is very difficult to describe exactly how overwhelming and awful depression can be. Trying to understand depression by remembering your own sadness is like trying to understand the sensation of drowning by taking a shower.

Depression
is a form of
self-sabotage
and I've done it
most of
my life.

But how did I really feel?

Depression, for me, is an overwhelming sense of loneliness. It starts with the belief that no one wants to spend any time with me, that no one really likes me and that the people around me just sort of tolerate my existence. Then it spirals down from there. Even if someone asks me to do something, I'll say no. I tell myself that with the mood I'm in, I'd be awful company anyway, so what's the point? I'd only bring everyone else down and they'd realize what a miserable, boring, negative person I am. Or worse, just how crazy I am. Then no one would invite me out again. Depression isn't rational, and it has this nasty way of making me try to prove that all the negative thoughts I have about myself are, in fact, true. My dad has always said that I like to make life harder for myself and he's right, but it's the depression – the imbalance within me – that makes me do it.

Psychologists identify typical patterns of distorted thinking which have a strong negative bias – Frankie is a good example of this, especially as she begins to feel hopeless very quickly.

Even now, when more and more people are opening up and talking about their own mental health, I can still feel cut off and apart. I envy people who have 'normal' thoughts and a laid-back attitude to life, people who can live life to its full potential of happiness. I feel like there's a cap on my happiness, like it can't quite reach its true height, no matter how much I want it to. It makes the lead-up to happy events really stressful because I'm scared that I won't respond in the right way or feel what I'm supposed to feel.

Frankie talks about a sense of emptiness and a lack of joy. This feeling is sometimes called anhedonia, a Greek word meaning 'without pleasure'.

Celebrations fill me with dread. The expectation to be happy, to have a smile on my face and be the life and soul of the party seems too overwhelming for my nervous system. I try not to think about it until it actually happens and I try to take a back seat in any plans in order to take the pressure off my anxiety, telling myself, 'It's one day out of the year. Does it really matter if you're not the life and soul of the party on that day?' I know the answer, but I get so preoccupied with not wanting to let anybody down. I also feel these situations only magnify the fact that I am never as happy or carefree as everyone else. Other people seem to find it so easy to let their hair down and enjoy special occasions, which ends up making me feel even more self-conscious and sad that I can't be more like them. And that leads to huge amounts of fear before big celebratory moments. I am so aware of the fact that my life doesn't warrant my sadness. I often feel that if it did, it would make it easier somehow.

Guilt is a big issue for me. It has a strong grip on my thoughts and actions and is something I battle with every day – which also prevents me from accepting the lows . The narrative of my guilt is always the same: 'I have been so fortunate to do the job I love and to experience all the things I have, so why do I feel such unhappiness?'

Guilt leads to feelings of sorrow, sadness and remorse. Frankie feels she needs to increase her guilt in order to appreciate what she has.

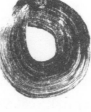
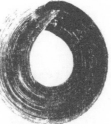

Here are some things I feel guilty about:

That I will never be the friend I wish I could be. The one who makes her friends feel how important they are, gives them all the time they deserve, celebrates their every achievement and is fully there for them through any hard times. I still have all my friends from home and I'm proud of that, as I've always had this notion that you can't fully trust someone who doesn't have at least one friend from their childhood – but my career took me away for long periods of time at a young age and, although I know they're all proud of me and will support me through everything, I do sometimes feel that it's hindered my chance to be the best friend I could be for them.

That I will never be able to fully show my children just how deeply and insanely love them. I will never be able to give them enough hugs and kisses, or tell them enough times how much I love them. I will never be able to give them all of me, my undivided attention. My biggest fear is that they will end up like me, with mental health problems. And if they do, I know I'll believe that it's my fault, like I've failed them by missing a sign, or missing something they were struggling with. I know I will tell myself that they would be happier if I'd done something differently, or if I wasn't their mum.

That I can never be the mum who remembers everything in my children's diary correctly, who is there at every sports day, doctor's appointment, sad day and great day. The mum who helps with all their homework, plans perfect parties, plays hours of endless games, is patient at all times and drops them off and picks them up every day from school, all while earning a living in order to give them everything I ever could.

That I can never be the wife I always imagined I would be. Loving, kind, fun and affectionate every minute of the day, who also runs the house and irons his shirts. The fact that, mentally, I have to be busy and have a separate purpose from my family fills me with guilt, but without work to focus on, I'm not sure who I am and what my purpose in life is.

That I have made mistakes, been selfish and run from my responsibilities at some points in my life. I was young when Wayne and I met, and I knew exactly what I wanted in life – to be a young mum and to get married. Wayne gave me all that, but I haven't always been grateful. I suppose I had a lot of my own growing up to do, while being a grown-up. I've never regretted a moment of being a parent and a wife, but it took me a while to give myself the chance to be good at it and stop telling myself I couldn't do it, or asking, 'What if?'

That I can't be the perfect work colleague because I am always doubting myself. I get so excited and passionate about a project, then spend most of my time trying to avoid it and telling myself I can't do it. My team have the constant task of picking me up, pushing me forward and convincing me that I can. They work so hard. I always feel there's so much more I should be, or can be, or could have done in my career, if only my brain didn't keep convincing me otherwise.

That I have caused sadness to my parents. My illness has forced them to question whether they had any part to play in it, and they have had to see me hospitalized because of it. I know that this has affected Mum, and she has definitely struggled with it over the years.

That there are people in the world living full and happy lives who die too soon, and here I am, wasting my chance at life, feeling sad all the time.

That my husband and children have a wife and mum with a mental illness and I cannot be emotionally and mentally there for them at all times.

These are what Cognitive Behavioural Therapists might call Frankie's 'core beliefs' and the way she talks about them shows the distortions in thinking that they lead to. She applies a negative mental filter, magnifying her faults and minimizing her contribution.

'Core beliefs' are a central feature of Cognitive Behavioural Therapy and therapists would encourage patients to challenge core beliefs and develop new, more adaptive core beliefs.

People who suffer with mental illness often worry that their children might develop it too and, for most mental illness, there is no genetic test or way of knowing what the risk to children might be. Fortunately, the evidence tells us that while genes are indeed important in a lot of mental illness, they are not the be-all and end-all. And medical science moves forwards, not backwards. The speed of diagnosis keeps improving and with each passing year we are researching more and better treatments for depression. I have a great deal of hope for Frankie, who is still a young woman, and even more for her children, or any children who may go on to get this illness.

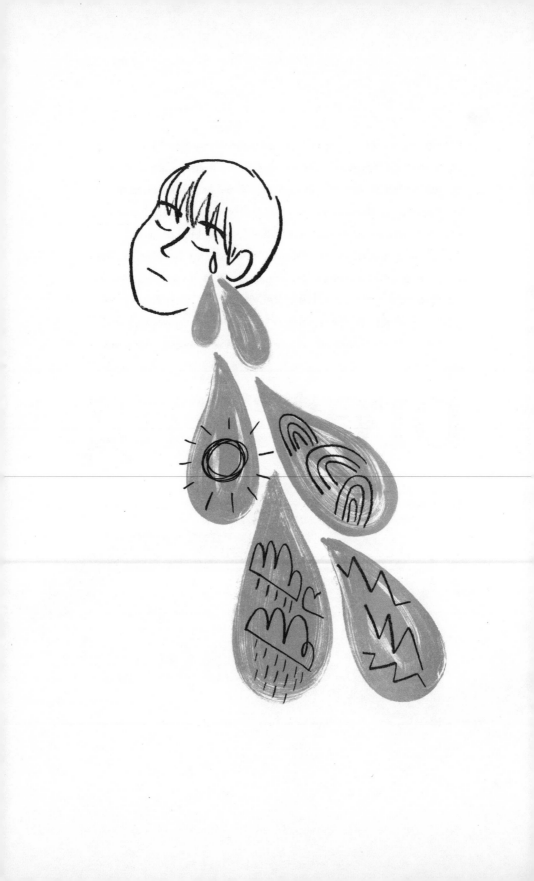

CHAPTER FOUR

breaking point

BREAKING POINT

Work has always been the easiest place for me to bury my head in the sand and avoid my thoughts. Other than being something I love, work is constant, busy and filled with a lot of other people telling you what to do. It's a place where I've never really had to think very much for myself or have an opinion or analysed my life in too great detail. I have a job that makes it very easy to become someone else and it has allowed me to run from the real 'me' rather than force me to confront myself. In fact, I'm not sure whether you have to be slightly crazy to be in my particular line of work, or if doing it makes you slightly crazy. Maybe it's a bit of both? It certainly has helped to distract me from nagging thoughts. Work was another coping strategy.

Frankie used work as an 'emotional anesthetic' – a temporary distraction from the way she was feeling inside. Work, especially work that is glamorous, varied or very busy, can successfully draw our attention away from what is going on inside by forcing us to focus on what's happening on the outside. There is an obvious trap, which is that working to the exclusion of sleep, rest, family and social life will drain, deplete and eventually exhaust us, leaving us wide open to the underlying depression. While we are busy digging in the garden, behind our backs the house is burning down.

Even with these coping strategies in place, it had got to the stage where I had started coming home and crying relentlessly again. Night after night, I would cry myself to sleep, then wake up in the morning, slap on a smile and go to work. It was totally draining. I remember sitting with Wayne in our kitchen and just sobbing uncontrollably, explaining that I hated my life and I couldn't handle being in the band any more. I was constantly exhausted from the hectic schedule and lack of rest days. And although we all have those bad days at work where you have to paint a smile on your face and get on with your day, for me it was becoming a constant, all-consuming daily task. I felt very little self-worth, my anxiety towards my body image was at an all-time high and the panic attacks were increasing at an unstoppable rate. I was reaching a tipping point.

Night after night, I would cry myself to sleep, then wake up in the moring, slap on a smile and go to work.

There's one day from this dark period that really stands out in my mind. We were doing a show with a meet and greet beforehand. As much as I loved meeting our fans, I'd started to feel like I was having to fight even harder to be the person they wanted me to be. I remember that for this particular day, I had to take a moment to myself, close my eyes and take a deep breath, to get myself into the role of 'Frankie from The Saturdays'. This shocked me. How had I got to a point where the two sides of my life no longer belonged to the same person?

Me.

I couldn't
find a way
to stop
myself from
falling.

Wayne said I should leave the band if it was making me unhappy and that we could cope financially if I wasn't working. However, deep down I knew quitting wouldn't fix anything, because it fed into so many of my anxieties; I'd be letting so many people down – the fans, the girls, management, my family, friends and, of course, myself. I would view myself as even more of a massive failure, and what would that lead to? How could I walk away from a job that so many other people wanted? That I had wanted for as long as I could remember. I think because my career started at such a young age, it became something that defined me and sculpted my identity in my own mind, too. I also knew that I had absolutely no idea who I was without my job. I'd been Frankie Bridge the pop star for nearly ten years already. I was the role. The role was me. It was a vicious circle; I couldn't live without it, but I certainly couldn't go on living with it.

It was clear that Frankie was caught between two powerful forces. One is her natural feelings of responsibility towards those who depend on her and who she has made a commitment to, the other is her own need to be needed. It takes considerable self-honesty for workaholics to see the obvious – that their whole identity has become that of someone who is valued and needed by others and that, without their work, they lack a strong sense of who or what they are.

It became clear to me and to those close to me that my plan to go it alone, without medication or therapy, really wasn't working. It was time to reach out for professional help again. We had a new manager by this time, and he suggested that I went to see the GP he always used with his artists. I made an appointment and was immediately referred to a psychiatrist, Dr Mike McPhillips.

I felt instantly comfortable with Mike. He was friendly and caring, but still so professional. Not only did he understand how I was feeling, but he also seemed as eager as I was to try to and find new means to make me feel better. He also fully understood my line of work and my need to be able to keep going despite my declining mental health. It was such a relief and I trusted him completely. He prescribed Sertraline for the depression and Alprazolam for the panic attacks.

Mike also referred me to Maleha Khan, a clinical psychologist specializing in Cognitive Behavioural Therapy (CBT), so I could talk everything through. I was hesitant at first, because talking hadn't got me very far last time, but I liked Mike and believed he knew what he was doing, so I agreed to give it a go. Before Mal and I met for the first time, I remember feeling that I had nothing to say to her and being determined that whatever happened, she wouldn't see me cry. I just couldn't face

My plan to go it alone, without medication or therapy, really wasn't working.

the idea of letting her in. Boy, was I wrong! She was so calm and genuinely seemed to care. She didn't talk down to me or treat me as just another patient, so I felt at ease. I talked non-stop – and cried quite a lot too.

And so a new course of treatment started, with first steps towards more progressive help. I was hopeful that it would, at last, help to ease my sadness, and that my life and mental health would turn a corner.

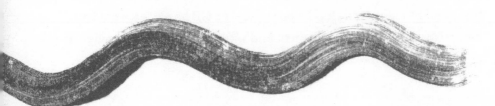

WHAT IS COGNITIVE BEHAVIOURAL THERAPY?

CBT has become one of the best researched, most widely practised and most effective forms of psychotherapy in the world. The original model has been developed and extended to treat other conditions such as day-to-day stress (mindfulness-based CBT), chronic pain (Acceptance and Commitment Therapy) and personality disorders (Dialectical Behavioural Therapy).

In CBT, the therapist and patient work together to identify and solve problems – it is a truly collaborative approach. It can help us think differently about ourselves and our past and teach us that we are not victims of our thinking and that we can certainly change the way we feel. This is not via reassurance or a 'pull yourself together' approach, but through understanding our thinking as this is what creates our uncomfortable and suffocating feelings. It works because we learn to change the way we think, feel and behave through thinking about our thinking.

CBT teaches us to question why we are allowing ourselves to think as we do, asking, 'Is it logical, is it rational, is it helpful?' And, crucially, it requires us to act differently.

One day, I had arranged to go and view a new house that Wayne and I wanted to look around. I'd taken the car into London and, because I wasn't used to the drive back to Surrey, I decided to follow the sat nav. I ended up on the M25 at rush hour. I knew I was going to miss my appointment. I felt so furious with myself. Although it was such as minor thing, it was also another example of just how useless I was. I felt as though I couldn't do anything right. I was such a failure and a let-down that I couldn't even make it home on time. I just sat in the traffic in my car and cried my eyes out. Hard, loud, uncontrollable sobs came out of me, like an out-of-body experience. I felt so numb – like I didn't have any particular feelings at all – yet at the same time, I was utterly overwhelmed and lost. What was the point of carrying on with life? Wayne was amazing and he deserved someone so much better than me. He deserved a woman who could at least perform a simple task like getting to a meeting on time.

I felt as though I couldn't do anything right. I was such a failure and a let-down.

I was completely engulfed by a sudden, strong urge to drive my car into the nearest wall, but as I was stuck bumper-to-bumper, I couldn't do it. The fact that I couldn't even manage to hurt myself made me angry. I was so disappointed in myself and at an utter loss as to how to go on. I remember thinking, 'You're a useless waste of a human being, do everyone a favour and put everyone out of the misery of having to deal with you.' But I was also aware that if I did kill myself, I'd be leaving behind so many people I loved, leaving them with so many questions and so much misplaced guilt. But how could I carry on?

Things just continued to escalate from this moment on. The constant crying continued. It was like my body had started working autonomously; I no longer knew how to control myself or my emotions. Wayne and I would plan to go out for dinner, I would go off to get ready, and then he'd find me either sitting crying in my dressing room, or asleep on the floor. I was exhausted. I was finding it too draining trying to keep it all together. It was at this point that I began shutting down.

One day, Wayne bought me the wrong food, and everything went from bad to terrible. I was so upset, I felt like he didn't know me at all. How could he get it so wrong? Clearly, he didn't love me and why would he? To me, in that moment, it confirmed what I already felt: I wasn't lovable. I wasn't worthy of anyone's love. Something so insignificant as a yoghurt brought on one of the biggest breakdowns in my life.

We had planned to go out for dinner that night. I really wanted to pull myself together and get ready, but I just couldn't. I broke down crying in my dressing room and, when Wayne came in to find me, I collapsed into his arms. He had to physically hold me up. I remember saying on repeat, 'I just want to die, I want to be dead.' In fact, the idea of dying terrified me, but it was the only way I could find to escape my thoughts. I couldn't think of any other way out.

Somehow, I managed to do what I'd always done; slapped on some make-up, chose an outfit, got myself out and drove us to dinner. In the car, I was quiet and grumpy, and Wayne told me to 'cheer up'. That sent me over the edge. I just screamed at him: 'How dare you! Don't you think I want to? If it was that easy, I would! Do you really think I want to feel this way, this unbearable sense of absolute misery?' He got out of the car, slammed the door and stormed off. I was in shock. How had my life reached this point?

I drove back to the house. How had I lost all control? This thing, this darkness, this 'Sunshine and Showers', this secret Frankie, this panicked person, this anxiety that I'd had control over for all these years had now taken complete control over me. I was broken and sad to the core; right down to my very bones. I had no idea who I was any more. I couldn't tell which thoughts were mine and which were caused by the depression. I just knew I couldn't go on. I was afraid of what thoughts I'd have next and I didn't trust myself not to follow through with taking my own life that night, or in the days or weeks to come.

Wayne eventually calmed down and came home. We talked it out, both knowing something needed to change. I needed help – we both needed help. Wayne couldn't be responsible for me or my actions any more than I could. It was clear that the medication I was on and the therapy I was having just weren't enough. But neither of us had any idea what to do. We were both scared of what was going to happen next, but knew something needed to be done.

Frankie's husband couldn't understand why she was so angry. Anger and irritability are known symptoms of depression, which is doubly unfortunate because, while we can all identify that someone who is crying needs our sympathy, anger pushes away those people who wish to help, or is met with anger in return, leaving us isolated from others just when we need them most.

The next morning Wayne rang my GP and she came over to the house. This wasn't usual practice, but she knew we were in a desperate way and that it was something that needed to be handled sensitively, properly and immediately. By this point I didn't know how to feel any more.

I'd been feeling
    so many feelings
    all at once
        for so long,
    that I had now
lost my ability
        to feel and
    my body
        had reached
    its final
    breaking point.

All I knew was that I wanted a life with Wayne, a life that was really worth living, rather than just existing from one day to the next. And I wanted children with him. I always had and it was something Wayne and I had discussed, but I knew there was no way I could bring a child into the world in the state I was in. At that point, I wasn't sure I would even be alive to see that day happen.

My GP made a few calls. She spoke to Dr Mike McPhillips and they both agreed that the only chance I had to get better would be to go into hospital. Over the past six months I'd seen two therapists and tried CBT, Prozac, Venlafaxine and Sertraline. By this point I was beyond caring what was done to me; I would have done anything just to feel anything remotely normal again. So all that was left was for me to find the time in my work diary. That was easier said than done. The Saturdays had a two-day video shoot abroad and it wasn't something I could just pull out of because so much time and money had gone into the planning and everything had been scheduled with precision. So we agreed that I would do the video and then come straight back and go into hospital. Luckily, our manager at the time had known me for years, as I'd worked with him in S Club Juniors too. He was caring and understood I needed help and was willing to do what he could to make sure I got it.

It was a relief to have a plan and to know that there were other people, apart from me and Wayne, who knew what was going on and how to help us both. The doctors explained that they felt hospital would be the best option because it was the only way for me to get proper rest and find the treatment I needed to get better. I had so many commitments that there would always be a reason to miss an appointment, or to keep working instead. It had to be something drastic that forced me to stop and focus 100 per cent on my health.

I look at the video we made before I was admitted to hospital now and I feel so sad for the girl I see on screen. The reason I don't say 'me' is because I don't see that girl and me, 'us', as the same person. It wasn't me. Yes, it was my body, but that was about it, she was a shell of a person. But when I look at that version of me, all I see is true sadness, a slight deadness behind the eyes. I was so thin then, too, and at the time I loved people telling me how thin I looked and how I'd gone too far. It made me feel happy, because it meant I was still capable of taking control, when I felt so out of control in every way. It's hard to look alive when you truly don't care whether you are or not.

It was a relief to have a plan and to know that there were people who knew what was going on and how to help us.

At one point during the filming there was a problem with the weather and there was talk of the video needing an extra day. I felt the panic inside me starting to rise. I had prepared myself for two days, just another 48 hours of pretending. I had built myself up, pushed myself to my absolute limit to get through it and I physically couldn't handle any more. My manager was the only person there who knew about my upcoming hospitalization, and so he knew how important it was for me to end on time. Luckily we managed to make it all work. Otherwise, I wonder if I would have managed, there was nothing left of me.

Wayne picked me up from the airport and it was such a relief to be back with him, back with someone who knew exactly what was going on, no more pretending. There were paparazzi there taking pictures of us walking together and it's funny, looking at the pictures you wouldn't have any idea of the pain, fear and sadness we were both feeling as it was locked away from their probing lenses. That's the thing about depression – it's good at hiding from the world.

I had decided not to tell my family about my stay in hospital. I just couldn't. The shame of having to admit to my parents and sister that my beautiful life wasn't enough for me, that I'd failed to function as a normal human being, that I found it all too much to handle. The idea of calling them and telling them something that I knew they would blame themselves for and would make them question their decision to let me go into the music industry was too hard to bear. I couldn't face any visitors either. I didn't want to have to explain myself. I simply had nothing left to give.

So it was Wayne who came with me to check into the hospital. He was my constant, the person who knew me inside out and who had seen me at my worst and most vulnerable. He made

By this point, I was so afraid of who I'd become and what I was capable of doing to myself that I just wanted someone to make it all go away.

me feel safe and loved. I couldn't have done it with anyone else. Our drive to the hospital was oddly calm. Obviously, I was nervous – I had no idea what to expect – but it was a relief to know that I was no longer ignoring the issue and that I was finally doing something about it. The only way from here had to be up.

It's a scary thing to take yourself out of your comfort zone and hand yourself over to complete strangers, but I was so ready to go into hospital. By this point, I was so afraid of myself, of who I'd become and what I was capable of doing to myself, that I just wanted someone – anyone – to make it all go away.

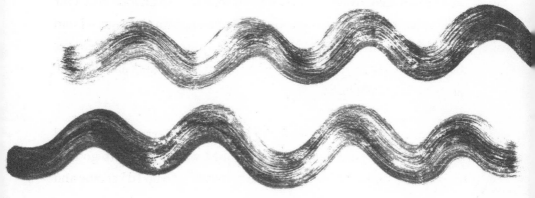

Here, Frankie is describing a very common emotional experience. At the point of dropping all of the pretence, there is often a wave of relief at not having to keep it up any longer. The emotional effort of doing so is simply exhausting.

OPEN NOTES

'Breakdown' is not a term that psychiatrists use very often, but it is a short way of saying 'I am unable to function in one of my key roles because of my symptoms', meaning that a person has left their job, or can no longer study, or has had to ask for help to raise their children, for example.

Admission to hospital is a rarity in the treatment of depression. It usually happens for one of three reasons:

- There is an immediate risk to life through suicidal thinking

- The patient needs a treatment that cannot be delivered easily to outpatients

- The patient can no longer cope with life outside hospital

In Frankie's case, it was largely the third of these that required her to go in. For some unlucky patients, it's all three.

Even if someone's condition doesn't involve hospitalization, it can be very difficult for their loved ones to understand what is going on.

The partners of depressed people may feel quite hurt that they are 'not enough' to keep a depressed person happy, but it is not a sensible way to look at the problem. You wouldn't expect loving someone to fix their asthma or diabetes for them because they are physical illnesses. So it is with depression.

One of the difficulties is finding ways to explain what is happening – either to loved ones or to others involved in the patient's daily life.

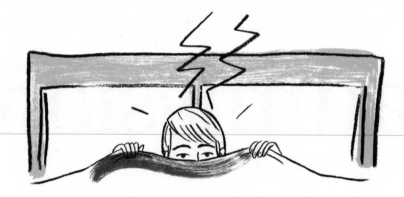

CHAPTER FIVE

admission

ADMISSION

All I knew about mental hospitals was what I had seen portrayed in the movies: padded walls and people chained to beds. In reality, it was nothing like that, except for the bit where everyone queues up to get their medication in those little paper cups. The rooms were very white and the chairs were all wipe-clean, but they were homely enough and I had my own bathroom. It was all surgically fresh and bright. The strangest aspect of the hospital was that I had in fact walked past it so many times before and had taken absolutely no notice of it, and now here I was living inside, as an inpatient.

I was diagnosed as severely depressed when I was admitted to Nightingale Hospital. I was crippled with anxiety, suffering from uncontrollable panic attacks, suicidal thoughts, constant tearfulness, poor concentration and paralysing negative thoughts about everything and anything. I had trouble sleeping, lacked energy and had lost my appetite and my libido. I couldn't do anything without help and was unable to function in everyday life. I couldn't fundamentally see the point of living any more.

They had to put me on new medication straightaway. The doses of Venlafaxine, Clonazepam and Diphenhydramine sleeping tablets were so high that my first few days in hospital are a blur. I slept most of the time as they needed me to rest before treatment properly got under way. I hadn't had a good night's sleep for so long, it was a relief to get some peace and quiet and to silence my mind so it could just switch off. It was all I wanted, not to think, not to be inside my own brain, locked in my own painful internal battle. An escape that felt almost impossible. For the first time, I realized why so many performers, or people in high-powered jobs, end up doing drugs – it's a way of getting the energy, the confidence and the mental capacity to do what's needed of them, and also frees them from their tormented minds.

I hadn't had a good night's sleep for so long, it was a relief to get some peace and quiet.

The next few days were focused on me trying to find my feet, experimenting with different medications and figuring out a schedule that would work for me. Mike came to see me every morning. It was always so nice to get his visits, something familiar in a very unfamiliar situation (although also bizarre because he used to cycle to work every day, so he'd always be wearing tight, bright Lycra and I'd only ever seen him in his office in pristine suits before), and, initially, we stuck to my private counselling sessions with Mal. I did a little bit of group CBT too, but I would get tired really quickly and easily, so I wasn't able to do much. I was nervous about sharing any of my issues with other people. Not because I felt I was famous, but because I felt that ever-recurring feeling of shame. I knew there would be people in there with worse problems than me, the child-star cliché. Also, my medication was so high that I was having very strong involuntary muscle movements (as if I didn't feel crazy enough already!).

Sadly, Frankie was in a bad way when she arrived, and it took a little time to find the right balance between not enough medication, which would leave her tearful, anxious and sleepless, and too much medication, which would leave her sedated and confused. The first few days in a mental hospital usually involve a lot of medical and nursing observation before we get the right balance.

Three days in, I decided to call my sister to let her know where I was. My mum answered the phone, so I had to 'fess up. I just told her very frankly that I couldn't cope any more and that I had decided the hospital was the best place for me, so that was where I was. Now I'm a mum myself, I realize how much it must have hurt my parents to find out such a big thing had been going on with their daughter without their knowledge.

A couple of friends have told me they came to visit me around this time, but I have absolutely no recollection of them coming or spending any time with them. Either I've blanked out a lot of things, or the medication meant I was too out of it to know what was going on. I do remember my sister coming. She visited as much as possible, but I never really had very much to say: she just came and lay in bed with me and watched TV. But it was nice just to have her close.

Wayne was a constant too, absolutely amazing throughout it all. Especially considering we hadn't been together that long and that a lot of my anxiety at this point was wrapped up in how my previous relationship had ended. Between training and playing football, he would come and see me whenever he could. He lost a lot of weight around this time, the lightest he's ever been. Now we think it was due to the stress of it all, but at the time, I didn't notice how badly everything was affecting him. Because I was in hospital, I didn't see the weight loss and I didn't see how sad and worried Wayne was in his everyday life.

So many people had experienced so many of the same feelings as me, if not worse, that I felt understood and not so alone.

As we've spoken about my breakdown over the years since, the stress it caused him has come out in both anger and sadness. I have understood more and more about how hurt he was and he has come to understand what I was going through and that it was nothing personal to him, us or anyone else around me. Learning all about this new illness and realizing that he couldn't make me happy was a lot for him to take on. And obviously, hearing about your partner's past isn't very enjoyable for anyone.

Once I had got my sleeping under control and I was no longer crying all the time, I started to integrate with the rest of the patients. We were a mixture of voluntary and admitted, and suffering from a range of illnesses from bipolar, depression and anxiety to Post-Traumatic Stress Disorder (PTSD), addiction and eating disorders. Everyone was so honest about their experiences. We openly discussed what medication we were on and why we were there. It was amazing, there were so many people who had experienced so many of the same feelings as me, if not worse, that I felt understood and not so alone. It was like a weight had suddenly been lifted from my shoulders. I no longer had to hide, cover up and lie about how I was. I felt more like myself than I had done in what seemed like forever. And I felt safe.

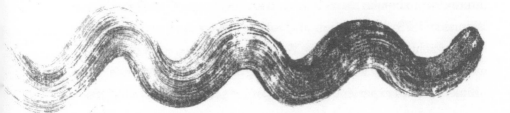

Being with others in a similar predicament makes a patient feel less isolated and meeting others with similar problems normalizes the experience of mental illness.

I had a fixed schedule which revolved entirely around getting me better and understanding myself more. I did art therapy, which I was rubbish at but enjoyed, I had a massage as often as I could – I know, pampered pooch – and a session where we had to sit in a group and say confrontational things to each other to provoke a reaction. I found that really hard as I've spent my life trying to avoid confrontation, but it was good for me to be encouraged to try it in a controlled environment. We had mindfulness sessions too, but I never got into that. It was too hard for me to sit and be with my thoughts and feelings. I couldn't clear my mind; it would just race even more and the anxiety would build until it was too much to bear.

Group therapy exposes people to complex interactions that are much harder to see in one-to-one therapy. The facilitator of the group is trained to observe and moderate the discussions, but people are usually very much themselves – introverts are quiet, extroverts over-share, compulsive helpers tend to become 'rescuers' and angry people usually express their inner rage. These interactions develop quite quickly and the group offers a mini laboratory in which patients can observe their own emotional responses to particular situations. This gives the opportunity to recognize faulty habits of thinking and acting and to practise better responses.

The practice of mindfulness wakes us up to the present moment and teaches us that the worries of our mental life distract us from actual life. In therapy, I would use mindfulness to help clients notice their urges. If we are mindful about their presence, we can then choose to either act on them, or learn that they can diminish. The client will learn to believe that if we don't act upon transient thoughts, urges, impulses, they will pass! Anxiety might initially increase, but it will plateau and then eventually pass.

I had started to make a couple of friends, which was a comfort; it's not recommended but of course you bond with certain people throughout your stay. There was one girl in particular and I just couldn't get my head around why she was there. She was absolutely beautiful; petite, dark-skinned with long, gorgeous hair. And she dressed amazingly. I always wondered how someone so beautiful could be so unhappy. Which made me realize that even someone who suffers with her own mental health can think exactly like so many in society, assuming beauty equals happiness.

Frankie is correct to say that we recommend caution when making friends in a psychiatric hospital. Most fellow patients are friendly and straightforward, but some may have complex personality problems, or undeclared problems in relating to other people, and may not be quite as they initially seem. Doctors, nurses and therapists are bound by a duty of confidentiality to their patients so we cannot say all that we know about patients without consent. Having said that, we carefully screen patients who we admit to a general psychiatric ward and there are separate hospitals that look after people who are truly dangerous to themselves or others.

There was one girl who frightened me a little bit too. She was on her fourth stay at Nightingale and had been admitted by the council. She wasn't a big fan of mine as I'd been moved into a bigger room that she clearly thought should have been hers. She would pace the hallways and talk to my visitors like we were great friends. She was totally convincing – they'd always be shocked when I told them we'd never actually had a conversation. She also shouted really loudly and got very angry when she realized I had a candle in my room, because it was against the rules. I had snuck it in, in the hope that no would notice. The smell just made me feel a little more at home. I suppose you could say she was the only one that fitted the stereotype of a 'typical' mental patient.

I also met a girl with bipolar disorder, an illness I knew nothing about at the time. I remember bumping into her in the hallway one day and she seemed so happy. She was pretty much bouncing around, really chatty and she explained that this was one of her episodes. I was almost a bit envious at the time, thinking how lovely it would be to feel that level of happiness; a level I don't think I've ever reached. But then, I never saw her mania crashing down either.

Another guy I became friends with had opened up in one of our sessions. He said his panic attacks made him feel like his back was ripping open. I'd assumed that all our panic attacks were the same and it amazed me that he experienced such different physical sensations. He also revealed that he'd completely planned his suicide. He had decided that he was going jump in front of a train. I felt so sad for him, that he had reached that point, but also, I found knowing that I hadn't gone that far in the planning of my suicide comforting.

I just wanted to find a way out of the place I had found myself in, not a way out of my own life.

I'd thought about suicide many times, but I had never actually worked out the details of how or when I would kill myself. Meeting someone who had done so made me realize that I didn't want to end my life after all. To most people, wanting to commit suicide and actually planning a suicide sound like exactly the same thing, unless you've actually had either of these thoughts yourself. The difference is although I had sometimes thought it would be easier to die, I knew deep down I couldn't follow through with it. Hearing someone who'd actually properly planned a suicide made me realize very quickly that they knew for certain that they wanted their life to be over and could have followed through with it, given the chance. But, in my case, I just wanted to find a way out of the place I had found myself in, not a way out of my own life.

Meeting others further along the road to recovery can be inspiring, and meeting others even less fortunate can be a consolation.

Being in the hospital also gave me time to rediscover things I was passionate about. My sister brought my guitar in for me so I could start practising again and Wayne brought me a box full of arts and crafts supplies, something I had always loved when I was growing up. It was an amazing feeling, almost childlike, to just sit and be me and enjoy doing something creative on my own and not being driven ever on by what was next on my schedule and the need to keep up the performance .

However, my eating was still very limited: it consisted of hot chocolate and chocolate digestive biscuits, but even this was an improvement. I had spent so long just getting by on adrenaline; my body was in a constant state of panic and anxiety. It meant that I had absolutely no appetite, and was always shaking due to the lack of sugar in my body. I think all the chocolate gave me the energy boost I needed, and it was easy to eat. Wayne brought me a big Christmas mug to use, so I had two of my favourite things in one! (That mug has always stayed precious to me. Silly, really, as the time when I was using it wasn't one of the best in my life, but that special connection to a small object makes me feel comfortable.)

As I had gone into hospital voluntarily, I was allowed to go on short outings, both alone and with friends and family. The first one wasn't a success. My sister and a family friend came to take me for dinner, but I couldn't make much conversation and my hyper-anxiety was in full swing. I found every simple decision really hard. Over and over, we would sit down in a restaurant, but it didn't feel right to me, so we got up and went somewhere else. However, the doctors thought it was good

In the
psychiatric
hospital,
I finally
had time
for myself that
I hadn't had
for years.

for me to get out, so we persisted. Pizza Express pretty much became my second home. It was familiar. I knew the menu, so there was no decision-making involved. My poor family probably had enough of it, but it quelled my anxiety.

I used to pop out for a walk around the shops by myself, too. It was so nice to be invisible, so good not to have anyone looking at me, not being on show. It's as if at some point in my life I lost the ability to make my own decisions, and lost confidence in them if I did, and these trips gave me time to figure out what I actually liked again and to rediscover my individuality and autonomy. After a few outings, I found I was actually capable of walking around a shop and picking things out that I wanted.

Therapeutic leave is a very useful tool. Not only does it cheer the patient up and keep them in touch with the outside world, it gives us a chance to identify challenges like the temptation to binge eat or to drink, or a problematic relationship with a particular friend or relative. Rehearsing a large range of daily activities is a good way for patients to discover whether they are ready to return to the outside world.

My dad and my grandad both had birthdays while I was in hospital. I didn't want to miss the celebrations, but they weren't easy for me. We all went to a Japanese restaurant in London for my dad's birthday. I felt so removed from the world and people around me and I still struggled to make conversation. It was a bit like being in a dream, I was there in body but not in mind. Being in a loud, busy place was overwhelming. It's weird when you feel like your life is stuck but for everyone else, the world is still turning and things are just carrying on as normal. Just being there was a big effort for me, so talking wasn't top of my agenda. My dad did manage to make me laugh, though. He had a pair of reading glasses with bright lights on either side so that he could read the menu in the dark. It felt such a shock to laugh but I was pleased that I still could and that some things were still funny.

My mum threw a big party for my grandad in Essex. I remember feeling really out of place and everyone commenting on how thin I was. I didn't feel I was the same as anyone else – no one else was currently living in a psychiatric hospital, dosed up to their eyeballs on medication, so it was hard to relate to any sort of meaningful conversation. I'd also started smoking in hospital (all the smokers got to go into the courtyard before bed, so I decided to join in and it helped to calm my nerves and ever-shaking body), and I snuck out for a cigarette during the party to calm myself down and take a break from all the noise and happiness. I found it so hard to be around happy people, partly because I didn't understand them and also because I was so envious then. Why was it so easy for them and not me? My mum came outside and caught me smoking. Smoking was a big no-go in our family and normally I'd have been gutted for her to see me with a cigarette, but at this point, I didn't care much about anything. Luckily, she just laughed and shook her head. Something that wouldn't have happened in any other circumstance, but given where I was, she was just pleased I'd managed to make it to the party at all.

Apart from these occasional outings, I didn't have much to do with the outside world and I certainly didn't go looking for stories online. However, my manager informed me that the press had been saying that I was in hospital seeking treatment for addiction. I couldn't really blame them – I'd assumed addiction was the only reason people went into a mental hospital too – but I found it incredibly frustrating and upsetting.

The press
　　coverage
made me realize
that
　　mental illness
　　　wasn't really
seen as a
　　genuine
　　　illness.

It's not that I didn't want people to think I had an addiction, as though that was something to be ashamed of, but it just wasn't *my truth*. It wasn't an important battle for me to fight at the time, but thinking about it now, it's probably what started me on my path of wanting to share my story and educate people about depression and anxiety. The press coverage made me realize that mental health just wasn't spoken about, certainly not by celebrities. It was something to be ashamed of and kept to yourself. I feel like people suffered in silence and just put it down to having a bad day – the good old British way of sweeping things under the rug.

Three weeks in and I had started to feel at home in Nightingale. I felt like I had my own flat in London and I had everything I needed. I suppose you could say I was becoming institutionalized, but the most important thing was that I felt safe.

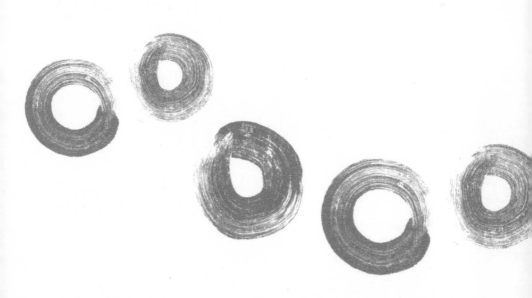

OPEN NOTES

Until a patient finds their feet in hospital, the visits and support of loved ones are crucial in keeping up their morale and in keeping a bridge open that leads back to the place they came from. At the end of their hospital stay, they will be walking back across that bridge, and we usually actively involve families, friends and even employers in planning a person's return to the community.

The patient will usually feel very guilty about asking people to go after they have taken the trouble to come, but visitors can be tiring. As a tip to visitors, little and often works best, and try not to overstay unless the patient asks you to remain. Do also check in advance with the nurses what time scheduled therapeutic activities and appointments are.

It's surprising how quickly a psychiatric hospital can become 'normal'. Patients and their relatives can be a little alarmed by this, fearing that the patient will become institutionalized. This is an understandable but hugely exaggerated fear. This is not something that happens to people who spend a few weeks in hospital. It is simply that they find the hospital a supportive environment in which they are free to say what they really feel. After spending time in psychiatric hospitals, as a patient or a member of staff, it can be surprising to observe just how much of the time 'normal' people do not say what they really think.

I don't think Frankie remembers this, but when I went to see her at the hospital for her sessions, she was very focused on leaving the group. She is so talented and has an interest in fashion and make-up, and she wanted to start her own brand. However, her lack of confidence in herself stopped her again.

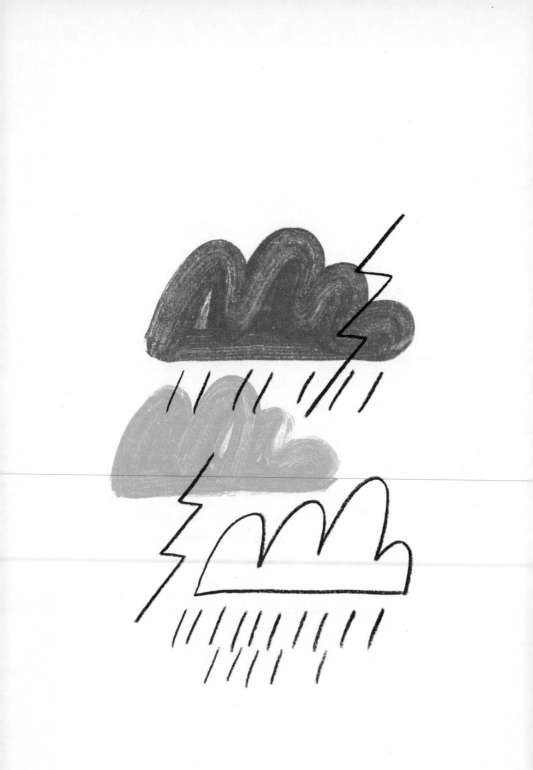

CHAPTER SIX

when will I get better?

WHEN WILL I GET BETTER?

My doctors had recommended that I should spend three months in hospital, but it became more and more apparent that that length of time just wasn't going to be possible due to external demands mounting up on me from the outside world. The band had already booked an arena tour that was due to start a few months after I was admitted, and the tickets were sold out. Touring was my favourite part of being a performer, as there was no better achievement than stepping out on to a stage and performing for the fans who had paid to come and watch us.

The doctors weren't convinced that going on tour would be good for me, but I was adamant. I had to be well enough to make it. I didn't want to let down the fans or the rest of the girls in the band. If I did that, I thought it would actually hinder my recovery and, besides, our insurance didn't cover mental illness so if I pulled out, we could be sued and find ourselves having to return a huge amount of money. That fear played a big part in my decision to carry on with the tour.

So, after four weeks in hospital, lots of plans were put in place for my discharge. I would continue my sessions with Mal twice a week, but in the comfort of my own home, and I would see Mike once a week too.

I would also have lots of private singing lessons to boost my confidence and take anti-anxiety medication an hour before each performance to try to contain my anxiety.

The doctors wanted me to stay closer to the centre of London so that my commute wasn't long and stressful. Luckily, Wayne had a house in Chelsea at the time, so we arranged to move there and asked the tour manager to pick me up and drop me off whenever I was working so I felt safe and comfortable. My work hours, including public appearances, publicity and rehearsals, would be built up slowly. I was also recommended some nutrient- and vitamin-rich shakes as a way of getting some goodness and energy into me as I was still unwilling to eat properly because of my perpetual fear of putting on weight.

I got a rush of fear, adrenaline and panic. It came out of nowhere and instantly overwhelmed me.

Two days after I was discharged, I went to do a gig in a nightclub. It felt right to step back into my 'normal' life and be back performing with the girls. I was miked up for rehearsal and ready to go when, all of a sudden, I got a rush of fear, adrenaline and panic. It came out of nowhere and instantly overwhelmed me. I just couldn't do it; I wasn't ready. The thought of going back to being 'Frankie from The Saturdays', in front of hundreds of people, just didn't feel possible. I burst into uncontrollable tears and dropped to the floor. The feeling engulfed me. My whole body went weak and I couldn't breathe. I was so frustrated that this was still happening to me – after all the therapy, the medication, the month in hospital, I was still unable to return to my normal life. The girls were scared; they had never seen me in this state before and didn't know what to do for me. I think it was a big eye-opener for them to see what I had clearly been hiding from them for so long. Our tour manager managed to get me into the car and back home. We would have to try again another day. I was upset at the time, but talking to Mal and Mike afterwards, I realized that what mattered was that I had tried. When you live with hyper-anxiety, you learn that trying is often better than overcoming it entirely.

Frankie realized that she was trying to run before she could walk. Most patients do a bit too much on leaving and learn to their cost that they have left the hospital as 'walking wounded'. I usually liken leaving hospital to leaving an orthopaedic ward wearing a walking cast on a broken leg – the bone has not yet fully healed and it will be months before the patient walks without stiffness and aching, much less going for a five-mile run. Frankie tried to do a gig 48 hours after leaving hospital and had a reminder that the underlying illness was still around.

The pressure was on, not only to be well enough to start tour rehearsals, but to be ready for a big TV performance in a few days' time. It was our first performance of our new single, 'My Heart Takes Over', live for *Children in Need*. I was determined to get through it, but it was easier said than done. Being back in my 'normal' life felt strange. The usual hustle and bustle in the changing room was overwhelming and suffocating and at one point it all proved too much and I had a panic attack in the toilets alone. Something that had been my everyday life for so long was now impossibly hard. But I'd worked so hard to get to this point mentally that I was determined not to let anyone down, myself included. And besides, we all got to wear long, sparkly gowns! I hadn't dressed up or had my hair and make-up done for ages and it felt great to feel a small piece of my old, shiny self again. Even if it was just on the outside.

The performance went perfectly. I was proud of myself for getting through it, but the negative voices had been swirling around my head the whole time. I was completely drained afterwards, physically and mentally. Watching the performance back, I looked confident and in control, but that façade couldn't be further from the truth. To be honest, the only thing I took real confidence in was my weight. I knew I was thin, too thin, but I thought I looked great. It's terrifying really, how we can pretend to ourselves as much as we can to one another.

With that performance under my belt, it was time to start rehearsing for the tour. We had dancers; guys we had spent a lot of time with in the past and who were a constant source of amazing, positive energy, so it was a lot of fun and it felt good to be back dancing. Dancing has always been my favourite part of performing and something I felt I was strongest at. I'm no professional dancer, but I love it and I've always found picking up and remembering routines pretty easy. But now I was finding it hard to keep my mind focused. The one thing I had taken such pleasure in now became a real struggle. It felt as though I had lost my ability to retain new information and hold my concentration for a long period of time.

When we took a break, the girls went out and got something to eat with the boys while I stayed behind and tried to force down my microwaved vegetable soup on my own. More often than not, I couldn't, and returned to the safety of hot chocolate. I hated the idea of eating in front of people, the pressure to act natural while forcing myself to swallow food.

I was also still smoking, something that the girls weren't aware of until they caught me sitting outside on the stairs, trying to light a cigarette with my ever-shaking hands. I can still remember seeing the shock on their faces – it was the first time that I realized how much they must have thought I'd changed over the past few months. The truth was I hadn't, of course; it was just that I was unable to hide the real me from them any more and I didn't have the strength to to go on pretending. The more time went on, the more new, strange and un-Frankie things they discovered.

By the time the tour came around, I was off my anti-anxiety meds, as the panic attacks had evened out and my mood was definitely improving. I was having weekly private vocal lessons to help with my anxiety about my voice.

Performing brings me so much joy, but it also brings me so much anxiety.

Again, this made me feel like I was learning and taking control of the situation. Being given tools by a professional to improve and understand properly how the vocal chords work gave me a little extra, much-needed confidence boost. I was just pleased that I had managed to recover in time, just enough to be able to make the tour and not let anyone down. I was also back doing the part of the job that I loved, which was the touring, the dancing, the costumes, putting on a massive production with a huge crew for our fans. Even I don't understand how I can love and hate something so passionately at the same time. Performing brings me so much joy, but it also brings me so much anxiety. And sleep was still a massive problem and it persistently remained one. I still couldn't quiet my mind enough to fall asleep and then stay asleep, often waking with nightmares about people in my room.

Sleep is one of the last symptoms of depression to come completely back to normal. I never regard people as being fully recovered until this too has normalized.

My low self-esteem and body-image issues were persistent, and showed no sign of disappearing – in fact, they were centre-stage in my thoughts. Not that anyone would have guessed: I was strutting my stuff on stage every night in tiny costumes, acting like the most confident girl in the world. I even remember one of my costumes was a dress with cut-outs either side of my stomach, from my ribs down to my waist. My manager insisted that I add some material to it because he thought revealing my jutting-out ribs would set a bad example to other girls. He was right, of course: I wasn't setting the right example. I don't want other girls to feel they have to be unhealthy in order to be happy – I clearly wasn't – but at the time, his comments only made me feel prouder of how thin I'd managed to get, and I felt angry that he was asking me to hide it as it had taken so much control.

I was also becoming frustrated when I had my weekly catch-ups with Mike over Skype. I had been out of hospital for a while now, and although I was still taking medication for my depression, I still wasn't fixed. I'd put in all this work and effort, but I still wasn't 'normal'. I felt let down, both by myself and by my doctors.

I remember in one of my appointments Mike asked me to fill out yet another BDI-II form. BDI stands for Beck Depression Inventory (it's named after the inventor of CBT, Aaron Beck) and it's basically a questionnaire designed to assess the current severity of someone's depression. There are 21 questions that focus on the typical symptoms of depression – such as low mood, pessimism, sense of failure, guilt, self-hate, suicidal thoughts, crying, social withdrawal, insomnia, fatigue, appetite and loss of libido – and for each one, the patient has to pick the statement that best describes the way they've been feeling over the past two weeks. For example:

• **I don't cry any more than usual.**	**0**
• **I cry more now than I used to.**	**1**
• **I cry all the time now.**	**2**
• **I used to be able to cry, but now I can't cry even though I want to.**	**3**

The questionnaire scores each of the statements on a scale from 0 to 3, and the numbers are added up to an overall score that helps the doctor figure out how severe your depression is.

The BDI is a widely used psychometric test, but I've always found doing it really hard because my mood very rarely improves enough to change my answers from one test to the next, which makes me feel as though I'm not improving or stabilizing. Mike knows now not to bother doing them with me, but in this particular appointment, after I'd filled it out and scored no better than the last time, I asked him if most people on medication ever feel 'normal', or if those with depression just have to accept that there is a level of happiness they will never be able to reach. I assumed his answer would be 'yes', but it wasn't. I was shocked. He said that out of all 600 of his patients, he currently only had two who had had to be hospitalized and that, once on the right medication, most people found their mood returned to normal. So you could say they were 'fixed' and brought back to life. That didn't really help to make me feel better.

The fact that Mike can't just 'fix' me, no matter how hard he has tried, makes us both pretty sad and disappointed. I have been one of his most complicated patients and he often has to remind me just how far I have come.

I am sure that I do not have to explain that I am not disappointed in Frankie, but I am certainly disappointed for her. Frankie is an endlessly patient and generous-spirited person, and I do feel a little guilty and sad that I cannot simply 'fix' her depression.

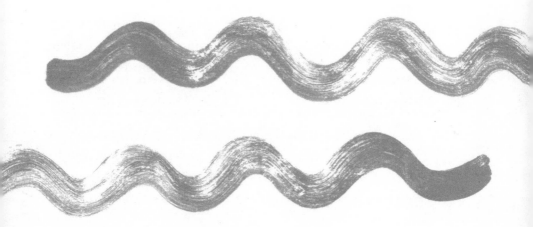

'RESPONSE TO TREATMENT' EXAMPLE QUESTIONNAIRE

Tests like the BDI-II forms that Frankie filled out are not a screening tool for depression; they are used to monitor the severity of the illness and the patient's response to treatment. Psychometric tests of this type can include questions similar to the ones on these pages, which are based on the PHQ9, a depression questionnaire commonly used by GPs in the UK.

Over the last two weeks, how often have you been bothered by any of the following problems:

Little interest or pleasure in doing things?

- ☐ 0 Not at all
- ☐ 1 Several days
- ☐ 2 More than half the days
- ☐ 3 Nearly every day

Trouble falling or staying asleep, or sleeping too much?

- ☐ 0 Not at all
- ☐ 1 Several days
- ☐ 2 More than half the days
- ☐ 3 Nearly every day

Feeling down, depressed or hopeless?

- ☐ 0 Not at all
- ☐ 1 Several days
- ☐ 2 More than half the days
- ☐ 3 Nearly every day

Feeling tired or having little energy?

- ☐ 0 Not at all
- ☐ 1 Several days
- ☐ 2 More than half the days
- ☐ 3 Nearly every day

Poor appetite or overeating?

- ☐ 0 Not at all
- ☐ 1 Several days
- ☐ 2 More than half the days
- ☐ 3 Nearly every day

Feeling bad about yourself, or thinking that you are a failure or have let yourself or others down?

- ☐ 0 Not at all
- ☐ 1 Several days
- ☐ 2 More than half the days
- ☐ 3 Nearly every day

Trouble concentrating on things, such as reading a newspaper or watching TV?

- ☐ 0 Not at all
- ☐ 1 Several days
- ☐ 2 More than half the days
- ☐ 3 Nearly every day

Moving or speaking noticeably more slowly than usual? Or being more fidgety or restless than usual?

- ☐ 0 Not at all
- ☐ 1 Several days
- ☐ 2 More than half the days
- ☐ 3 Nearly every day

Having thoughts that you would be better off dead, or of hurting yourself in some way?

- ☐ 0 Not at all
- ☐ 1 Several days
- ☐ 2 More than half the days
- ☐ 3 Nearly every day

OPEN NOTES

Most of us don't want to be ill at all, much less have an illness that's going to interfere with our ability to lead a normal life, so when we do get ill, the first question most people ask is, 'When will I get better?'

While this is a sensible question, the one we should in fact ask is, 'Will I get better?' For any given person with depression, there is roughly a one-third chance that the answer will be yes, a one-third chance of significant improvement and a one-third chance that initial treatment will not be successful.'

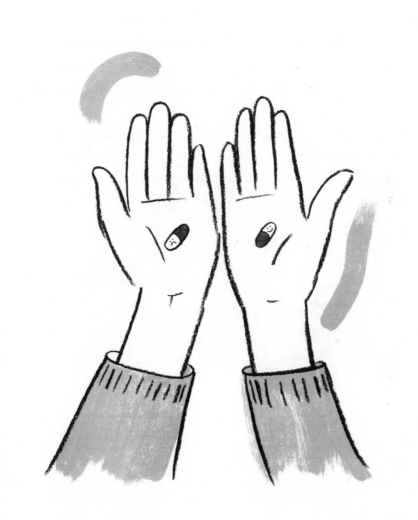

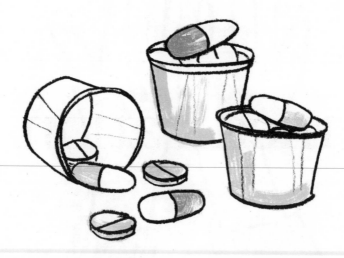

CHAPTER SEVEN

medication

MEDICATION

Without medication, I don't think I would be here today. Don't get me wrong, it wasn't a quick fix and it certainly wasn't an easy ride, but it has definitely taken the edge off my depression. Medication has been a controversial subject for so many years and that's something that needs to change. We would never raise an eyebrow at someone taking insulin for diabetes, or an inhaler for asthma, so why are people more comfortable talking about Viagra than antidepressants or 'happy pills'?

Medications used to treat anxiety and depression are among the most frequently prescribed drugs in Europe.

I believe this is down to people having to openly accept that they aren't happy, and that their life is less than perfect. Or perhaps it's the fear that, due to people's poor understanding of mental health illnesses, they will be viewed as mad or unreliable. I've definitely overheard conversations where people talk about someone else and judge them because they are on antidepressants, as though they have failed to be strong in some way. I've even had friends who have lowered their moods massively and suffered awful side effects by taking themselves off their medication suddenly because they've been fed the cultural myth that you can't stay on antidepressants for a long period of time. Why not? If they help you to live your life better and enable you to function in everyday life, then what is the embarrassment? *Where is the shame in medicine?*

Equally, I get very frustrated with doctors who just stick people on antidepressants, without giving them the full picture and without properly checking whether medication is right for that particular person's problem. A friend of mine was put on them without being given any idea of the possible side effects, or the complications of coming off them. And they didn't improve her mood. She eventually stopped taking them, and had two rounds of therapy and felt a million times better. All she needed was someone to talk to because her depression was circumstantial, not chemical. That doesn't make it any less serious, or important; it just needs to be treated differently.

The majority of patients believe that therapy is the cure-all treatment. They are encouraged to do so by the media, which encourages people to believe that if they discover an underlying conflict in their mind then, with the help of a therapist, they will be fully cured of their condition.

There is also a general sense that medication is like putting a sticking plaster over the problem, rather than really getting to grips with it, that doctors are trigger-happy when it comes to prescribing and that therapy will provide lasting benefits that will keep a person well in the future, whereas medication will stop working as soon as the patient stops taking it.

Often, these things are true: therapy is the best approach and it really does provide benefits for the future once it ends.

However, this is most true of a comparatively mild depression with an easily identifiable trigger and a recent onset. Sadly, Frankie's illness is not mild and she came to therapy in a very deteriorated state, with her worst-ever symptoms. There are several factors in her illness that strongly suggest she should be on very long-term medication:

- First, she was young when her illness first began and has a family history of depression, both of which suggest a strong genetic influence
- Second, there was no clear and obvious trigger for her episodes
- Third, she has shown little tendency in the past to go into spontaneous remission, her illness simply grumbles away for year after year
- Fourth, though she has found therapy very helpful, it has never been enough on its own to keep her well
- Fifth, her illness is both disabling and dangerous; it has the capacity to stop her in her tracks and put her in a psychiatric hospital for months at a time

For Frankie, long-term preventive medication is presently a reality that she has come to accept as the price of living a full and normal life uninterrupted by breakdowns.

My own journey with medication has been long and frustrating. And it's still ongoing. Mike has reached the conclusion that I have Treatment

Resistant Depression. That means I seem to respond well at first, then slowly the medication becomes less and less effective, even though I always end up taking the maximum dosage possible – often the same amount recommended for a large man (sometimes twice the size of me!).

The side effects are often the problem too. Typically, the medicine results in headaches, nausea, tiredness, low – or no – libido, a horrendously dry mouth, weight gain, constipation and, most embarrassing of all, involuntary muscle spasms (although, in truth, none of them are great!).

Depression is usually defined as being resistant to treatment if it has failed to respond to two different antidepressants given for an adequate time period (usually at least 6–8 weeks) and at adequate doses (at, or near the top of, the recommended dose range for each drug), with good compliance (meaning that the patient has been consistently taking the medication) and with no other obvious complicating factor (such as heavy drinking or drug use). Treatment Resistant Depression affects up to 30 per cent of my longer-term patients.

For Frankie, the most commonly used modern antidepressants either did not work, or ceased to work. The older medications, which we have turned to now, commonly had side effects, no matter how carefully we used them. There is great interest in new treatments for depression, some of which have come along since I first saw Frankie. One, which is actively used at the Nightingale Hospital, is Repetitive Transcranial Magnetic Stimulation. This is a very well-tolerated treatment that consists of 20-minute sessions of applying a targeted magnetic field to the area of the brain that governs mood.

At the moment it has been approved by the National Institute for Clinical Excellence (NICE), but it is not widely available because of the cost. A familiar story.

Day-to-day life with anxiety and depression is hard enough already, so these side effects clearly don't make things any easier and when you're hoping the medication is going to fix you, they are really hard to accept. The dry mouth makes singing and TV work more difficult, the weight gain contributes to my depression and anxiety and my low libido has been a recurring issue in my relationship. I totally understand why – joined with my self-loathing and low confidence, it's not the sexiest combination. It must be very hard for Wayne to accept that my lack of interest in sex is because of my medication and has nothing to do with my feelings for him, or how much I am attracted to him.

We have tried all sorts of concoctions:

- **SSRIs (selective serotonin re-uptake inhibitors).** Thought to increase serotonin levels in the brain, these are mainly prescribed to treat depression, particularly persistent or severe cases, often in combination with a talking therapy. They have fewer side effects than most other types of antidepressant, so are often the first choice.

- **SNRIs (Serotonin and norepinephrine re-uptake inhibitors).** These are similar to SSRIs and were designed to be more effective. The evidence for that is uncertain, but some people seem to respond to them better.

- **Prozac.** This is a type of SSRI and often used to treat depression,

Obsessive Compulsive Disorder and bulimia. It tends to have fewer side effects than other forms of antidepressant.

- **Sertraline.** Another type of SSRI, this is sometimes used to treat panic attacks, OCD and Post-Traumatic Stress Disorder, as well as depression.

- **Bupropion.** This antidepressant is sometimes used as an add-on with other first-line treatments such as SSRIs when there has been no, or only a partial, response.

- **Buspirone.** This is an anti-anxiety medicine used to treat physical symptoms of anxiety, such as fear, tension, irritability and dizziness.

- **Venlafaxine.** This antidepressant is sometimes used to treat anxiety and panic attacks, as well as depression.

- **Mirtazapine.** This antidepressant is used to treat depression and also sometimes OCD and anxiety disorders.

- **Duloxetine.** Another form of antidepressant used to treat depression and anxiety.

- **Imipramine.** Mainly to treat depression, this antidepressant can also reduce symptoms of anxiety.

- **Lofepramine.** One of the oldest antidepressants on the market, this has more unpleasant side effects than more modern forms. It is only prescribed if other types of antidepressant have been ineffective.

If you are on antidepressants, you will not float through life with a big smile on your face no matter what happens to you.

- **Clonazepam.** A type of benzodiazepine tranquilizer, this acts to produce a calming effect on the central nervous system and is used to treat panic disorders and specific types of seizure disorders.

- **Xanax.** Another type of benzodiazepine tranquilizer, used as an alternative to Clonazepam.

It's a pretty hefty list, especially as I don't rely solely on medication to do all the work. I have spent – and continue to spend – hours of my life in therapy too, because I believe the two should always go hand in hand. I also try to keep up my fitness as much as possible, and do my best to stay open and honest about my thoughts and feelings with everyone around me so that I don't slip back into old habits of concealing and internalizing my pain and suffering. The problem is, I don't want to always be a burden, or the person who's forever bringing down the mood.

Mike once described medication to me as 'like a life-jacket that will keep you bobbing along if you fall in the water and stop you sinking'.

It's stuck with me because it just made perfect sense in my life.

The medication I take makes my life livable and manageable. I still have my ups and downs, my good and bad days, but it stops me from slipping back into that deep, dark hole. Basically, it stops me from having another mental breakdown and ending up back in hospital.

Ultimately, I have to adopt the belt and braces method as I know it will keep me afloat. I know how lucky I have been financially to be able to pay for my treatment. I wouldn't have been able to afford my stay in hospital at the time without Wayne's support and I will always be truly grateful for that. I also had private healthcare that helped pay for most of my therapy sessions, and now I pay for them myself as and when I need them. I know this won't be the case for everyone and that the wait for treatment on the NHS can be a long and frustrating. Don't let that put you off. You will get there and it's well worth the wait.

The most important thing is for you to find what works for you. It will be different for everyone as no one has the same story, chemical make-up or imbalances. The truth is you have to try lots of things in order to find out what helps you and supports you throughout the day. But remember, you are on the right track, even if things can feel a little bumpy at times when you are trying to navigate the often confusing landscape that is mental health. You have taken the most important step and are on the way towards finding what helps you – whether that is asking for help from a friend, speaking to someone, going to your GP or taking medication.

Do what feels right for you today.

OPEN NOTES

Antidepressants are not 'happy pills'. They do not take away normal emotional pain. If you drop a hammer on your toe, you will yelp with pain, and if someone close to you dies, you will grieve. What antidepressants often will do is prevent a massive and disproportionate illness being triggered by an upsetting life event. I compare them to a life-jacket: wearing one won't stop you falling off the boat and if you do, you will get wet and the water will briefly close over your head. But you will bob back up to the surface. You will not sink to the bottom.

Most depressed patients are to some extent agitated and anxious, and most severely anxious patients suffer low mood. They are closely related conditions and they often occur in the same person at the same time. Even the treatments are similar. However, anxiety can be quickly relieved by sedatives, whereas simply taking a Valium will not actually treat depression. Sometimes it is only when we have relieved the symptoms of anxiety that a patient realizes how profoundly sad they have been.

A good proportion of depressed patients are given sleeping tablets and sedatives in addition to their antidepressants so that they can relax, make use of therapy and sleep well enough to keep functioning while they are waiting for their antidepressants to work. At that point the sleeping medication can be tapered off.

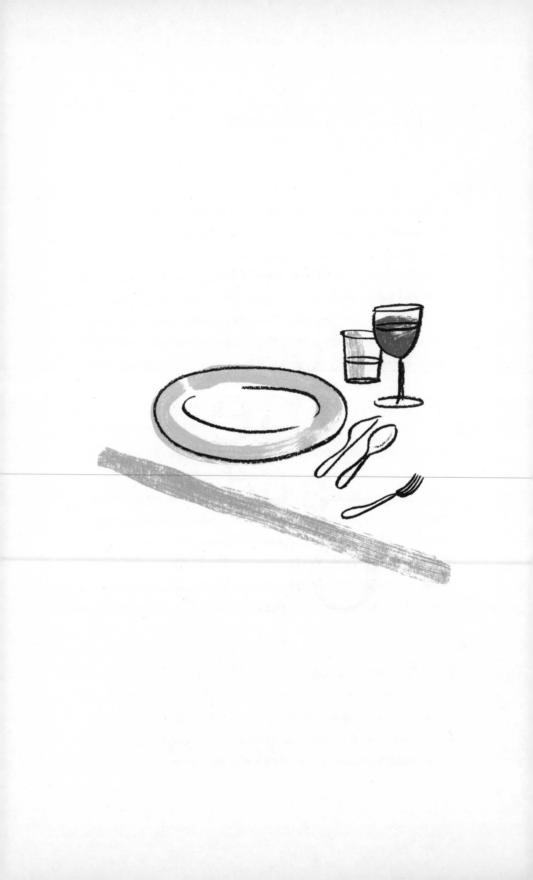

CHAPTER EIGHT

food, me and OCD

FOOD, ME AND OCD

I've had a difficult relationship with food for most of my life. It started when I was a child: I was a really fussy eater, afraid to try new things and terrified that I'd eat something that was going to make me sick. But it became more about control as I became an adult. It seems that eating disorders are yet another symptom of my depression and anxiety, a fact that I have only recently come to accept and understand. The two are linked. When I am up, I eat. When I am down, I don't.

As my mental health deteriorated, my relationship with food took a turn for the worse. It was a lot easier to hide as I got older and was preparing my own meals. Because work was so hectic, we ate most of our food on the go, so I rarely sat at a table with other people and no one really saw what I ate or how much I often didn't. I found comfort in controlling what I ate and very quickly that became a habit I wasn't even aware of, or a coping strategy I realize I had built in order to restore some power over the world I existed in, rather than feeling rendered powerless by my mind. Eating wasn't something I ever enjoyed doing, it never seemed like an important part of my day and certainly wasn't a priority. I avoided carbohydrates like potatoes, bread and pasta and eventually no longer craved them, simply eating whatever was quick and gave me an energy boost. I hated the thought of a full plate and would always make a point of leaving something. It felt like a victory not to finish a plate of food and to go to sleep feeling hungry. Full-fat Coke was a staple of my diet, and if that didn't do the trick, there was always a granola bar near by. It was ironic, really, as both are full of sugar, but I didn't eat them in large enough quantities to affect my weight and they gave me just enough energy to keep going and never gave me the feeling of being 'full'.

It seems that eating disorders are a symptom of my depression and anxiety. When I am up, I eat. When I am down, I don't.

At my lowest, I thought that the people others said looked ill and too thin looked better than I did, so it made me feel powerful if anyone ever told me they thought *I* looked too thin. Trying on clothes that once fitted me and finding they were too big or seeing my collar and hip bones sticking out felt like an achievement, allowing me to think that perhaps I was good at something in life after all, even if that was punishing myself with hunger. It spurred me on to create even more restrictive habits. And it was something else for me to be able to concentrate on, a distraction from everything else that was going on in my mind. I felt I was such a horrible person on the inside that the one thing I could control was my outside appearance – what people saw when they first looked at me. If I could make this perfect then people wouldn't figure out what actually lay within.

People with eating disorders and body-image problems fall into the trap of thinking everything is about food and that happiness is found by simply eating less of it, or getting rid of it once they have eaten it. The lightbulb moment here is to realize that food has become a channel into which every difficult feeling is directed. A huge range of stressors and disappointments will therefore come to act as triggers to starve, binge, purge or exercise, as though these behaviours would somehow make us feel better about loneliness or exam nerves or being let down by someone. These things have nothing to with food and it is bizarre to imagine that acting dysfunctionally with food could successfully medicate these feelings. The food trap is simple but deadly. It is almost never actually about the food, but we try to pretend that food is the answer.

I have come to understand that a lot of my eating issues were driven by my anxiety and my need to exert some sort of control over my life. However, being in the band certainly didn't help. The beginning of The Saturdays was particularly hard, as we were all trying to find our roles in the group, not as a collection of individual women. A girl group is not the same as a band of musicians where there's the bassist, drummer, guitarist and front person. We were essentially all equals, yet we all knew that wasn't entirely true – it was pretty clear from the beginning that I wasn't going to be one of the main singers. I understood why – most of the girls had incredible voices and I was happy to accept that mine wasn't quite as strong – but it did leave me wondering what my role was exactly in the group dynamic.

Once the band started to pick up some success, I quickly learned the real reason that I was there was for what I was wearing and who

I was dating. Being someone who has always loved performing, it was a painful realization. Although I got lots of attention which, at first, soothed my worry as people were interested in me, liked the way I looked, saw me as a role model and cared about what I was up to, after a while, the constant scrutiny of my life choices and how I looked became a pressure that I found too hard to handle.

For the first few years, I refused to change and people seemed to like that I wasn't the 'typical' girl band member – I had a bit of an edge to my style, my choice in music, my short hair. But over the years my confidence in that wavered and I became increasingly self-conscious about every aspect of who I was and how I presented myself. I started to become overly self-aware, and began to question every little thing about myself and my life.

We all compare ourselves to other people in our everyday, 'normal' lives, but being in the band, five girls together every day, made it much worse. If one of us lost weight, it spurred the others on to want to do the same. Each of the girls had something I envied and because I had accepted the fact that singing wasn't going to be my selling point in the band, I put all my efforts into my appearance and I decided that I looked best when I looked thin.

○

Frankie was falling into a trap of anorexia, which is a life-threatening illness with the highest mortality of any psychiatric disorder. The condition has been on the increase for both men and women, and people can suffer with anorexia for their whole lives. There are both biological and psychological factors behind the onset of anorexia. Women with a first-degree relative (a parent or sibling)

suffering from an eating disorder have a tenfold increased lifetime
risk of developing one themselves, and people with perfectionistic,
obsessive personality traits are also more susceptible to the disorder.
Psychological and sociocultural factors include perfectionism,
helplessness, inability to cope with stress, rumination and worry
and competitiveness and comparison within peer groups.

After a while I wasn't even aware that I was restricting my food because
it had become my new normal. It became the way I lived, not a way I had
to live. That's the destructive thing about eating disorders. I didn't really
see until I fell pregnant and discovered I had a proper appetite how
abnormal and unhealthy my diet had become. Once I had got through
the morning sickness, I began to enjoy food and looked forward to meals
for the first time in my life. It's a feeling that's continued ever since.

Of course, I know it's healthy that I now enjoy
food, but I find it frustrating too. My size still
has such a huge effect on my mood and when
I become aware that I'm feeling down and less
confident, my go-to is to work on my weight.
I am careful now though and exercise rather
than limiting my calorie intake dramatically.

My starving technique was a coping mechanism and another way to escape my sadness.

What often happens when people feel sad is
they then inflict more sadness on themselves
through punishing themselves. My starving technique was a coping
mechanism and equally another way to escape my sadness – the less
I ate, the less I could mentally be totally all there. The truth is deep
down I was mentally unwell and my illness told me that I was a horrible
person. I didn't want anyone to find out, I wanted to keep up the Frankie
charade. The charade I had done for my whole life. Not eating became

part of keeping the real me from view and making myself small made me feel stronger. Thinking back on it, I feel sorry for the person I was, I was unwell and trying to do anything to cope.

It used to be easy for me to avoid food – in The Saturdays, we were so busy that there were often days when I didn't eat anything – but these days it's almost impossible not to eat. A lot of my social life revolves around food and obviously I need to feed the boys every day. Also I'm at home more and when I get bored or tired, I eat. Something that I find frustrating now is that my old thoughts about food and my size are still there. Sometimes I still want to have that same sense of control that I used to have and I still want to be 'too thin', but my willpower is not the same as it was. Maybe that's because I'm in a better mental state? I now have more important things to think about, like my kids and my husband, bills and the mortgage. My low days come less often and they're not quite as low as they used to be. The sad thing is that I sometimes find myself wishing I was still the same as I used to be. But I know now that it's wrong.

OPEN NOTES

There are a variety of different eating disorders:

- **Anorexia.** Sufferers fear putting on weight and over-evaluate their shape and weight. They keep their weight down by restricting food and/or over-exercising and often behave in a ritualized way around food.

- **Binge eating.** This is the most common form of eating disorder. Sufferers regularly lose control of eating, consuming large portions of food, often in secret.

- **Bulimia.** Sufferers will overeat, as with binge eating, but then take compensatory action such as purging or using laxatives.

- **Orthorexia.** An obsession with eating 'pure' foods, orthorexia is not yet recognized by the American Psychiatric Association, but it is seen in clinical settings. The symptoms are eating very little food, exercising too much, spending a disproportionate amount of time worrying and obsessing about food and becoming preoccupied with body shape.

Obsessive Compulsive Disorder

I have also battled with OCD. I don't remember having it as a child (although I was convinced that if I couldn't picture a scenario in my head then it wasn't going to happen – for example, if I couldn't 'see' our plane landing, it meant we were going to crash), but as I got older and my depression and anxiety increased, I started to develop all sorts of obsessions. I turned numbers into a digital-clock format in my mind, I counted how many individual lines made up a word or number and how many steps I took on each floor tile. I avoided the cracks in the pavement, I counted the spaces between the street lamps when I was driving and, when I walked anywhere, I always made myself start with a certain foot.

I still have it today. My latest form of OCD involves cleanliness and worrying about germs. I don't clean excessively, but I can't relax in certain public places. It started while I was in The Saturdays, when I went through a phase of carrying plastic cutlery with me everywhere we went. We stopped off at so many service stations and I just couldn't trust that the knives and forks had been cleaned properly. The texture of the cutlery become a real issue for me too – I couldn't bear the feeling of the thin, tinny metal, or a slightly bent prong in my mouth. Even writing about it now gives me the shivers.

When we go on holiday, a rented villa is pretty much my worst nightmare, because I worry about whether the last people who stayed there washed the cutlery properly. Public toilets are an obvious problem, too. These anxieties mean that I spend a lot of my time on holiday or out in certain public places tense and unable to relax – literally cringing inside. It has got to the point where it takes the joy out of things that should be fun and I find it very frustrating.

It took me a long time to admit to Mal that I had OCD. I'm not sure why; out of all of the things I had told her this was probably the least personal. But to me, it seemed the strangest and the most complex. Even though it was something I did so often, I knew that there was nothing to gain from it and couldn't explain why it happened, so I felt ashamed. My OCD manifests itself in so many different ways, constantly changing the way it works, shows up and returns. I have had times when it feels like OCD is overshadowing all my thoughts, but I've learned to live with it. I know these thoughts are bred from my anxiety and I've taught myself to recognize them as a sign that my mood is slipping.

Ask for help and start to talk to someone about your OCD openly.

Practise mindfulness.

Listen to your fear and sit with it. Consider where it is coming from: is it from your mind or is it an outside threat?

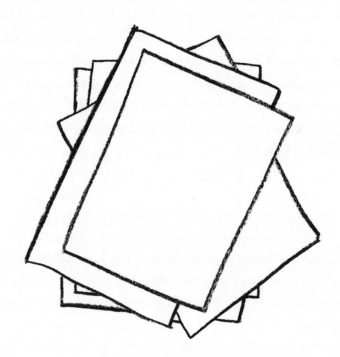

OPEN NOTES

Although psychiatric conditions like depression, panic attacks, anxiety, phobias and Obsessive Compulsive Disorder do happen in isolation from each other, it is not at all uncommon for a patient to have more than one of these conditions, and it is clear that there is some sort of link between depression and other anxiety-based disorders. Most psychiatrists believe that as our scientific understanding of the brain increases, we will understand the genetic basis of these links and use that knowledge to develop more effective treatments for them.

Obsessions are characterized by recurrent intrusive thoughts, images and impulses. These cause doubt, triggering the potential for danger which the person believes they have caused and can also prevent. Compulsions are actions or reactions, directly and meaningfully related to specific fears and are intended to prevent the imagined danger occurring. They are referred to as 'Neutralizing', as they are performed to remove the anticipated danger. They can include Overt Rituals, such as washing and checking, and mental corrections known as Covert Rituals.

OCD is not an entirely unusual phenomenon and can be reported by almost all of us at some point. People with intrusive thoughts are often shocked and terrified by those thoughts and feel a sense of responsibility for any harm that might happen as a result. This leads to them creating a series of behaviours designed to prevent any harm. However, since the compulsion is entirely unrelated to the intrusive thought, it has no effect and, as the person repeats the pairing again and again, the 'solution' becomes the problem. This can have a negative effect on the person's life and cause significant distress and disability.

The only effective treatment for OCD is Exposure and Response Prevention: the person is exposed to their fear – contamination, for example – and then prevented from using an overt compulsion such as hand-washing to neutralize it. In the short term, this treatment causes the person's anxiety to rise but, before long, the brain realizes that there is no real threat to fight or run from, so the Threat Response in the brain calms down. Repeated exposure results in the anxiety easing until it eventually disappears.

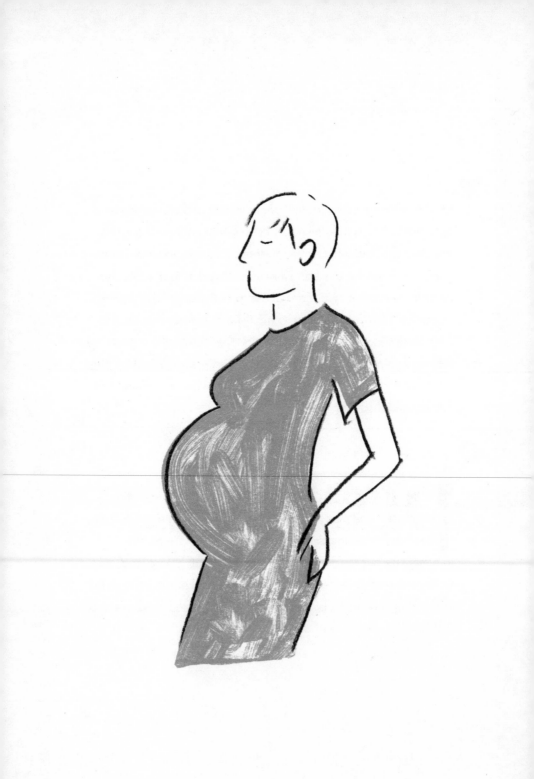

CHAPTER NINE

being

pregnant

BEING PREGNANT

I'd known my whole life that I wanted to be a young parent. Starting my career at such a young age made me grow up a lot quicker and I had to decide what I wanted out of life much earlier than most people. I knew having the perfect career and being comfortable financially wouldn't be enough for me in the long run. Consequently, I was always paranoid about letting my career completely take over my personal life and ending up at an age when children were no longer an option. And I liked the idea of being a young mum with enough energy to keep up with my kids, even as they got older. I was also aware that Wayne, being older than me, didn't want to wait much longer to start a family.

A year or so after my stint in hospital, I discussed the idea of having my own family with Mike. I was still on medication, a mixture of antidepressants and anti-anxiety medication, if and when it was needed. I was keeping up with my therapy on a regular basis. I wasn't fixed, but I had come a long way and felt ready.

I was done with going out and, having dedicated most of my life to my career, I felt I was ready to take that next step. Mike seemed to think I was in a strong position mentally to handle it and that giving me someone else to concentrate on could only be good for me. So Wayne and I decided to start trying. Una and Rochelle had already had babies, so I wasn't too nervous about telling the girls about our plans. I hadn't wanted to be the first band member to be pregnant, because we were still so busy and I didn't want people to panic and think it was the beginning of the end of The Saturdays. And me being me, I was too scared to be the first one to rock the boat. Luckily, all of us in the band had the same view that family was just as important as the music and so we always made it work.

I got pregnant very quickly. Wayne was away for a game when I did my first pregnancy test. I couldn't even call him as he was on a flight for

I liked the idea of being a young mum with enough energy to keep up with my kids, even as they got older.

the next few hours, but I needed to share my excitement with someone. Luckily my sister was at my house so I told her the news. You spend all this time hoping to get pregnant, then the day you find out that you are, everything changes but at the same time nothing actually changes at all. I started imagining what the baby would be like – boy or girl, fair, dark, a personality like mine or like Wayne's?

I had so many questions. But I didn't feel any different and there was no bump. So, while the biggest thing in my life had just happened, there was nothing to show for it.

I hadn't given it much thought before I fell pregnant but now the baby was in there, I realized there were only two ways to get it out, and I was terrified of both options! Natural birth scared me because there's no guarantee of what's going to happen, or exactly when the baby will be born, but a Caesarean seemed too clinical and surgical. Being cut open, awake...Not to mention all the needles involved in both scenarios.

I really started to worry about the medication I was on, too. I've always been aware that people say you can't take antidepressants while you're pregnant but I was terrified of the idea of coming off my meds. I went to see Mike as soon as possible and he reassured me that everything would be fine and he would monitor me as closely as possible. He told me that I wouldn't be able to take any of my anti-anxiety meds, but that the antidepressants I was on were safe to take throughout pregnancy. I was so relieved. We decided that in my position, the benefits outweighed the risks. I would be no good to a newborn baby if I ended up back in hospital and that's what we felt would happen if I was to go entirely medication free.

Taking medication throughout my pregnancy felt like such a taboo.

But still, taking medication throughout my pregnancy felt like such a taboo. Obviously, only certain things are safe to take while you are pregnant and it's advisable to talk to a specialist to decide the best plan of action and do what you feel is right for you and your family. But taking medication shouldn't be something that anyone should be made to feel ashamed of. Years ago it probably wasn't possible, but today, within reason, it can be done. Fortunately for me, Mike, Mal, my GP and my obstetrician all stayed in touch throughout my pregnancy and monitored me and my baby together, ensuring that we were both staying well.

It's a common misconception that women cannot take antidepressants during pregnancy. Even as recently as 20 years ago, medical students were being taught that pregnancy is such a happy time in a woman's life that she is somehow protected from depression, and that post-natal depression was a sudden and dramatic event caused by the hormonal changes and sleep problems that followed the delivery.

I would estimate that I have now treated well over 60 women through their pregnancies, and I am relieved and happy to say that there have been no cases of complications during or after the pregnancy and no need to hospitalize any treated patient for depression. Obviously, that is only one doctor's viewpoint and evidence on safety needs to come from very detailed research looking at tens of thousands of pregnancies, but the research that we do have is very encouraging and supports the choice of taking antidepressants throughout pregnancy if the woman's history of depression merits it.

My morning sickness started to kick in at around six weeks, which wasn't ideal. Doctors always say it's a sign of a strong pregnancy, but every time someone said that, I wanted to punch them!

I was trying to work my usual hours and keep the pregnancy a secret until I was ready to announce it and dance around without being violently sick. For me, the only way to ease the nausea was to eat. Anything beige would do – crisps, chips, bread, plain biscuits, all washed down with full-fat fizzy drinks. All the things I had spent half my life avoiding. I gained weight fast, and I also was suffering from water retention. By the time I was 12 weeks pregnant, I couldn't see the bones in my ankles and I was struggling to wear my normal clothes and shoes. I felt so out of control of my body and, in truth, I hated it. I had never been over eight and a half stone, so the change in my body really affected me. Carrying on working meant being seen by the public, when all I wanted to do was hide. I tried to find costumes that would fit in with what the other girls were wearing but that didn't make me look like I was trying to cover up and disguise my body. Standing next to girls who were all size eight every day and knowing I was growing bigger was a battle. The pressure to maintain a perfect image was quite high. Dancing felt silly, I didn't feel like me, so doing the same routines just didn't feel right. I was sure that everyone spent the whole performance laughing at me. I was well aware that the public had only ever seen me look a certain way and that this new look was as big a shock for them as it was for me.

> **I felt so out of control and so unlike myself, I was lost.**

The combination of the weight gain, constant nausea and tiredness really started to take its toll. I felt so out of control and so unlike myself, I was lost. At a time when I finally had everything I'd always wanted and should have been at my happiest, I found that I couldn't enjoy it in the way that I thought I would, and should. However, at the same time, I was aware of how magical it all was too. Every time I felt a kick or saw a scan with the baby wriggling around inside me, it reminded me of what I was doing all this for – to have my own family, a little piece of Wayne and me.

What I found really strange was talking to other women. They would always say how amazing being pregnant was and how much they loved it, but when I told them how hard I was finding it, their stories would change. It was as if no one was being honest about pregnancy. I was so shocked at how hard it was because no one had ever told me truthfully the toll it takes on a woman's mind and body. It's like an unspoken rule that you can't get pregnant and not enjoy it. For me, pregnancy was a means to an end – the beautiful little baby. I didn't have to love every second of the bit in between. It's the same as when you go on holiday: 90 per cent of the time, the travelling is a bit rubbish, but you have to do it to reach the awesome place you want to visit.

To make matters worse, I wasn't only dealing with my own opinion of myself, I was having to deal with the public's opinions and criticisms too. It was like any negative comment about my appearance was proof that I had been right all along. I spent a lot of time crying over what people were saying about me online. Throughout every public appearance, I felt apologetic for being there. Ashamed of the person I had become, embarrassed by the audacity I must have to still class myself as a member of a girl band.

This is another clear instance of Frankie battling with her Negative Automatic Thoughts (see also page 52). In depression and anxiety these thoughts may appear reasonable, but in fact, the more we listen to and believe them, the worse we feel.

It made me realize that while I've always been self-conscious about the way that I look, I also used my body as my armour. I didn't actually know who I was without being a size eight. I felt exposed and vulnerable. But as the saying goes, the show must go on! So that's what I did (minus the slutdrops!).

Whether you've been pregnant or not, you will undoubtedly have heard about the immediate, all-engulfing love that women feel when their baby is born. Instead of seeing this as something to look forward to, I just saw it as yet more pressure and something that I would undoubtedly fail at. I was terrified. What if I didn't love him straightaway, like everyone else did? What if I didn't feel like the baby was even mine, because when you think about it, you don't get to choose, do you? You just get what you're given. I was convinced that I would fail at one of the most significant parts of being a mother and mess this little newborn up from the moment he was born. Why do

I was terrified. What if I didn't love my baby straightaway, like everyone else did?

we place so much pressure on ourselves? We are already performing the everyday miracle of working while also growing a baby!

On top of that, there was the anxiety about post-natal depression. I was convinced that it was inevitable for someone who had a history of mental illness and had always struggled with depression. Surely I wouldn't be spared that?

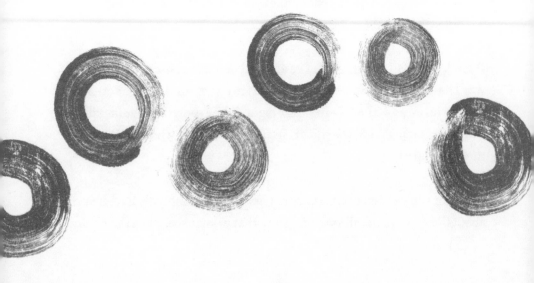

I don't
do well
in situations
where a certain
emotion
is expected
of me.

🌱

I share this concern with patients who have a severe history of depression. There is little about the realities of pregnancy that would prevent a person from becoming more anxious and depressed, and there is evidence that a lot of post-natal depression actually begins pre-natally and is only identified post-natally. We now believe that antidepressants protect against both ante-natal and post-natal depression – another example of the 'life-jacket' (see page 149) in action.

🌱

We now know that depression is quite common in pregnancy (occurring in around 10 per cent of all pregnancies), that it is especially common among women who have a past history of depression, and more common still among those who are already pre-natally depressed. The best way to prevent post-natal depression is to systematically identify and treat pre-natal depression. For this reason, along with all the other safety checks in early pregnancy, we are now screening pregnant women for depression.

I was so distracted by all my other anxieties that I didn't have time to overthink the C-section. It was a strange choice for someone who is terrified of death, pain and needles, but I felt a C-section was a more controlled environment. My obstetrician could tell me roughly what the procedure was, I had a time and a date and a good idea of what was going to happen. This helped me to feel more at ease. The thing I was most worried about was not being able to eat or drink in the lead-up to the operation! I was totally relaxed until the anaesthetist began to explain all the risks. It wasn't until he mentioned that sometimes the spinal block doesn't work properly and you can feel them inside of you that the anxiety and heavy breathing kicked in. From the moment the C-section was booked in, I had been asking my obstetrician what he does if someone freaks out on the table, and he always said no one ever does. I just kept thinking, well, probably no one has ever been as anxious as me, so I'll be your first.

On the day, I was due to have my first baby I was as calm as possible, and my only anxious moment was when I couldn't feel myself breathing due to the anaesthetic, and the uncontrollable shakes that took over my body.

The birth itself was not what I had imagined – I could hear the surgeons, elbow-deep inside me, talking about picking their kids up from school, while I was going through this monumental moment in my life. The normality of their conversation actually took my mind off my baby's imminent arrival. And the impending pressure to love him.

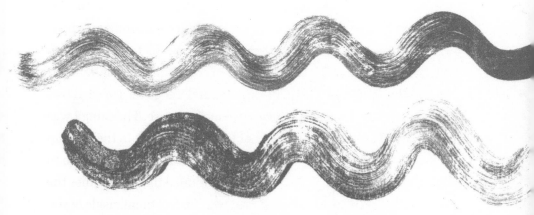

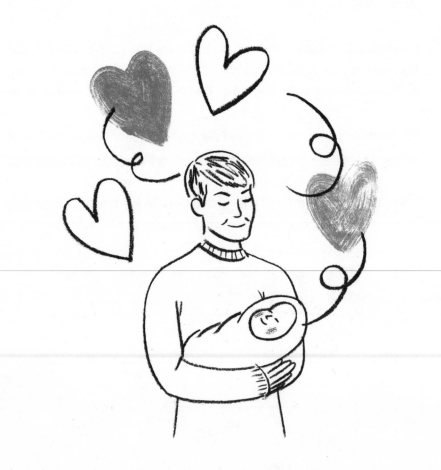

CHAPTER TEN

motherhood and me

MOTHERHOOD AND ME

I fell in love with my son the moment he was born. It was such an overwhelming rush of emotions. Suddenly he was there, perfectly formed and tiny. (He had always been so big in my mind while I was pregnant that I was convinced he was going to come out the size of a toddler.) I had no idea what the surgeons did to me after he came out, all I could think about was this little bundle of newness in my arms. That overwhelmed me and the world around me.

However, I want to be clear that although, yes, I did love him, no doubt about that, my love also grew with time. I think every new mother needs to give herself less of a hard time about the famous 'first flush of love'. You've carried this baby around inside you, done everything you can to keep it safe, given up parts of your life for the past 40 weeks, and possibly before that if you've been trying for a long time to conceive, and that continues in many different ways once it's born. Just because the baby is out, you don't suddenly have your old body back, you're not getting much sleep, whether or not you're breastfeeding, your life completely changes and at first they don't give much back in terms of responsiveness. Newborns are cute, but they are also hard work and the smiles and giggles don't start for a while, so give yourself a break if it takes a little longer for the love to really grow. (The same goes for new dads too.)

As I had decided to take antidepressants throughout my pregnancy, Parker had to be checked for a few days after he was born for withdrawal symptoms. I wondered once if the nurses were judging me, but I soon forgot to worry about what they thought of me. I couldn't take my eyes off him. Finally I had done something that I was ridiculously proud of. No amount of sold-out tours, best-selling singles and albums, or money made could beat this feeling. I just wanted to cuddle him all the time, he was all mine, I made him. The nurses offered to take him for a bit so I could sleep, but I liked having him where I could see him – or I did until he choked on some mucus, that is. That's when my anxiety kicked in. I hadn't thought about the dangers of mucus, I didn't think choking would be an issue until he was up and about and able to put things in his mouth! After that, I made the nurses take him while I slept, in case I didn't hear him choke in my sleep. The reality was starting to sink in: the responsibility for keeping my baby alive rested entirely on my shoulders.

He didn't start crying until we were driving home from hospital a few days later. I stuck my finger in his mouth for the whole journey. It was the only thing that seemed to make him stop. After that, it seemed like all he did was cry. I didn't know any different so I thought it was normal until I had my second baby.

I found it really stressful not being able to soothe him, as yet again it reminded me that I seemed never to do anything right and failed at everything. Wayne was amazing, he'd take him off and calm him down, no questions asked. I remember one night just crying and telling Wayne how terrified I was. People tell you all the time how strong your

My love
for this child
was almost
suffocating,
I felt it like
a physical
weight.

love for your children is, but although I love so many people in my life, I never understood how different it could be.

The fear of anything happening to my baby or him being the slightest bit unhappy hurt me physically. It was a feeling stronger than anything I have ever experienced in my life.

I hadn't originally put too much pressure on myself to breastfeed. I figured I would give it a try and go from there. Wayne had always said if he was a woman he'd choose a C-section and formula, so it was a relief to have no pressure or expectations from him. I quite liked breastfeeding my baby; it felt good to be doing absolutely everything I could for him, he just seemed to get what he was doing and it felt like a nice moment between us. However, after a few weeks I began to find it stressful and isolating. I wasn't one for whacking my boobs out in public and it just became a fight between Parker and me. Looking back, I now realize that I was engorged – my breasts were too full, so he had nothing to latch onto. He was hungry and crying, I was stressed, feeling like I'd failed him because I didn't know what was wrong and was also crying!

The thought that I was the only one who could feed him, that I was solely responsible for his nutrition, was beginning to bring back those pangs of anxiety. I wanted to be able to share the load. When I gave Parker his first bottle of formula, I was filled with guilt. I felt like I was giving up and basically feeding him poison. Fortunately that feeling didn't last long as he guzzled it down and seemed pretty content afterwards. I felt a huge sense of relief that I could now share the responsibility for feeding him. Unfortunately that didn't last long either, because Parker ended up with reflux and colic. He seemed so uncomfortable and constipated all the time, and after going backwards and forwards to the doctors, we finally got a diagnosis: he was allergic to the protein in cow's milk. This was something I had never heard of and I instantly felt awful, because he wouldn't have suffered so much if he had stayed on breast milk.

Although I now had new anxieties, all my other ones seemed to quieten down. It was like my mind was now too full of worry for Parker and I found I had no time or space for anything else. Suddenly, other things just didn't seem as important. Bringing another human into the world really puts things into perspective. I very quickly realized that I couldn't control everything that happens in the world. Seeing a baby try new things on a daily basis, having to let him figure things out and to accept that he will fall down sometimes gave me a new sense of freedom. Seeing life through a child's eyes forces you to appreciate the smallest of things, like the happiness

I very quickly realized that I couldn't control everything that happens in the world.

that bubbles can bring, or jumping on a trampoline, or even just the sight of your face in the morning. As much as the responsibility was overwhelming, it gave me a sense of purpose and meaning that I hadn't ever felt before. I have always made polite excuses about my professional success – I was lucky, in the right place at the right time and so on. I'd never acknowledged or taken any pride in the hard work and sacrifices I had put into achieving that success. It was the same with my friends and relationships. I just assumed people tolerated me. But being a mother was different; I knew he wouldn't be here without me and we needed each other equally. It was an amazing feeling. Turns out I'm quite needy and I thrive off feeling needed.

The weight I had put on while I was pregnant was coming off slowly. I'd found a trainer to help me get back in shape and she had put me on a safe and healthy diet and I was working out regularly. But it was slow going – too slow. Something just wasn't adding up, so one day she asked for a list of the medications I was taking. She did a lot of research and it turned out that in the cocktail of antidepressants I was taking, there was one with a lot of links to weight gain and water retention. Now it was all starting to make sense.

Weight gain is a common problem when managing a depressed patient in the long term. Unlike other side effects, which are usually obvious from day one, weight gain on medication is usually quite slow and it can take a long time to realize what is going on. Most women hate to gain weight and a lot of women struggle particularly badly after having a baby for all the obvious reasons: breastfeeding, disturbance of daily routine, reduced exercise and altered mealtimes.

I decided to do completely the wrong thing and stopped taking my medication immediately. I lost a stone in two weeks, but I felt horrendous. I was bedbound for days, totally incapable of getting up. I just sat with a bowl beside me, feeling horrifically nauseous, with the most excruciating headaches. The side effects didn't disappear, no matter how many painkillers or over-the-counter anti-sickness medications I took. I realized I should have consulted my doctor before coming off everything in one go.

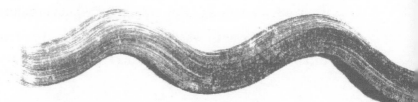

A good many patients do simply stop medication without getting a
withdrawal reaction, but in Frankie's case it did not work out, and
sensibly, she came back to see me to discuss a gentler way of stopping.

So I went back on the medication and asked Mike to help me come
off it properly. I reduced my intake slowly, lowering the dose a bit at a
time each week. The side effects were much more manageable – I was
prescribed anti-sickness medication to help ease the nausea and I had
paracetamol on hand all the time for the headaches – and, although
it took a few weeks and wasn't an enjoyable process, it was totally
worth it for the end goal of losing some weight. I did my own research
and couldn't believe the number of people who had suffered the same
problem. After that, the weight started coming off easily and I started
feeling like my old self again. I know it shouldn't have bothered me so
much, but I wanted to send a message to every single person who had
said horrible things about my weight gain and tell them exactly why it
had happened during my pregnancy.

Returning to work after having Parker wasn't too hard, I think because
I was still so in the thick of it with The Saturdays – I knew no different and
the other girls had done the same. Sad as it sounds, I was more worried
of about going back on stage still feeling overweight. I remember
doing my first performance post baby. I had already lost quite a lot
of weight, but I was nowhere near the size I was before I had Parker.
I got a message online from a girl saying she couldn't believe I had
the audacity to be on TV looking that fat. I was incredibly hurt,
it had taken so much courage to get back up on that stage and
she'd said exactly what I was already insecure and worried about.
I couldn't believe it and it felt humiliating for all my internal worries to

be voiced in public, as though my inner critic was right and I was being exposed to the outside world at a time when I felt my most vulnerable and defenceless.

When Parker was about 18 months old, Wayne and I decided to have another baby. I knew The Saturdays were winding down and I was coming to the last few weeks of *Strictly Come Dancing*. Doing that show had given me a big confidence boost that there was life for me without the back-up of four other women. Parker was at a really cute and easy stage, so it seemed like a good time to start trying. I knew I wanted Parker to have a brother or sister and I had always wanted them to be relatively close in age. It also meant I had more time at home to really enjoy having a newborn. However the guilt of 'ruining Parker's life' was very strong for me. He had been the apple of my eye and I was afraid he'd feel abandoned, or that I wouldn't love the new baby as much as my first. Feelings that are perfectly normal for most second-time mums.

On the day I was supposed to start rehearsals for the *Strictly Come Dancing* tour, I started being violently sick. It was constant and never-ending. I couldn't even pick myself up to make it to the toilet in time, so I just sat in our bedroom with a bucket at the ready. I was gutted about letting Kevin Clifton, my dance partner, down but I was convinced I would be back in the studio the next day and able to carry on as normal. But my body had other plans. The sickness continued and when I called my obstetrician and described my symptoms, he broke the news that I was suffering from hyperemesis. It's a rare condition in pregnancy, characterized by severe nausea and vomiting. He explained that there was no way I would be capable of doing the rehearsals, let alone the tour because the more tired you get, the worse the symptoms are. So I had to pull out of the tour, citing my pregnancy as the reason.

I was devastated. I was disappointed about not being able to dance again and about letting everyone down and I was also terrified of what people would say. Fortunately, however, Kate Middleton has been very open about her experience of hyperemesis during her pregnancies, so people were actually very sympathetic about it. I was completely bedbound. I couldn't even bear to be around anyone else – just the smell of another person was enough to set me off. It was a surefire cure for my sickness phobia, but I felt I was abandoning Parker before the new baby was even born.

In truth, I felt as though I had brought this on myself. When I first found out I was pregnant again, I was happy but also petrified of putting on all the weight I had worked so hard to lose, so I told myself that this was my punishment for having an ungrateful, selfish thought at such a magical moment. (Although my sickness meant that I started my pregnancy by losing half a stone!) After a few weeks I was prescribed some anti-sickness medication that took the edge off and meant I could just about function again. Eating beige food, little and often, seemed to help.

We should all just do what's right for ourselves and our babies.

This time, I managed to put on two stone instead of four. As I was now on an anti-depressant that didn't affect my weight, and as I wasn't working as often nor doing many performances with The Saturdays, the normal weight gain of the pregnancy didn't affect me quite as much. I didn't feel as 'on show' and, to be honest, I was just happy to be able to move my eyes without being sick. I think having been so horribly ill at the start of this pregnancy meant that when the sickness finally calmed down, I enjoyed the experience slightly more. I played around with different maternity outfits, had a few changes of hair style – that kind of thing. But let's not get too carried away. I was still painfully self-conscious.

Once Carter was born, Parker didn't seem particularly fazed by his existence. He was so young himself, I don't think he really understood. I decided to breastfeed Carter for four weeks, because that's what I did for Parker and that way my guilt-addled mind felt less to blame. However, it didn't go to plan with Carter; his latch wasn't great and he was cluster feeding for three hours at a time with only an hour's gap between each session. I just used to sit and sob. I felt like I was doing exactly what I didn't want to do. I was abandoning Parker.

We decided to get a night nanny. I was beside myself when she arrived, so I just handed Carter to her and begged her to help me. She got me pumping and it turned out that one breast produced half as much as the other so he was never getting a full feed. Immediately, it all seemed so simple, but it was something that I would never have been able to figure out on my own. I had spent so long feeling like such a failure, yet it turned out there was nothing I could have done.

Breastfeeding is absolutely natural in as far as we have breasts to feed our babies and our bodies produce milk, but that doesn't mean either mother or baby immediately knows how to do it. Unless your baby is magically born with the knack or you have someone to help you who knows what they're doing, it can be bloomin' hard! So give it a go if you want to, but no one should feel a sense of failure if it doesn't work. We should all just do what's right for ourselves and our babies. Make sure to confide in your friends, and in other mothers. Everyone has different motherhood ups and downs.

The important thing is to find what makes you a happier mum, as it make for a happier baby too.

Although I still question every single thing I do and worry about it, having kids has made me more confident in my own opinions and decisions. It has taught me that I can actually handle a little confrontation if needed for the sake of my boys. In fact, I once faced up to a woman on a flight back from a holiday who had turned around and told me to 'control my naughty child'. I was furious. It probably wouldn't have bothered me so much if he was being a nuisance, but he wasn't. I told her how rude she was and said she should get a private jet if she couldn't handle the public around her. I was crying and shaking by the end, and I definitely shouldn't have sworn at her, but I was proud of myself for standing up to someone. It was a first. Motherhood had changed me. It had helped me stand up for my children and for myself too.

Becoming a mother has taught me that I could protect my family. I would fail at times but I would do everything in my power to keep them alive. Motherhood has also helped me to live for the smaller moments of joy and appreciate every one of them. And, most of all, it has taught me that I am stronger than I think I am.

I have
reserves of
inner strength
that nothing,
not even
my illness,
can take
away from me.

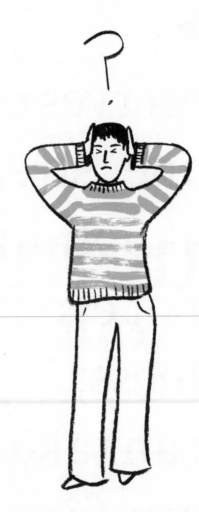

CHAPTER ELEVEN

tuning
out

TUNING OUT

One of the biggest changes to my life and to all our lives has been the introduction of social media into every part of our lives. As someone who has had the same career for the last 18 years, it's been quite an adjustment to create and manage a social-media persona as well as my public one and private one too. Back in 2001, when I first started in the industry, social media didn't exist. I was unaware of what people thought of me and I only shared what I chose to in front of the cameras at work.

When The Saturdays formed in 2007, online forums were just beginning to become popular and we were asked to sign in and interact with fans. It was fun but also quite intimidating, because while it was lovely to get to chat to our fans directly, having to encounter some of the not-so-nice conversations was really hard. Back then we weren't expected to do much, and we didn't have to get too involved on a regular basis. We would just sign in to the forums as and when we wanted, usually before or after a show, send a few replies to a handful of people and sign out again, so weren't prey to everyone and anyone's opinions of us.

Then news websites appeared. This is one of the parts of my job that I still have a love–hate relationship with. We need each other. Online news is an immediate, constant and hugely successful way for your face and name to be instantly seen by millions of people. When the story is a good one, you're buzzing; but when it's something negative, it stings. Then there's the reader feedback in the comments section. I used to read all of the comments and let them destroy me. I would convince myself that if this was one person's opinion, then it must be everyone's. We were always told not to look at the comments, but I've always said that's like telling someone, 'Behind that door there's a room full of people all talking about you, but don't put your ear against the door and listen.' It's impossible. Once you know the comments are there, you can't stop yourself from looking.

However, one day I did just that. The story about the actor Paul Walker's tragic death in a car accident was all over the internet. I wondered what kind of comments people would write. I was so shocked at the disgusting and disrespectful things people said. It made me realize that if people can write awful things about a young man who'd just lost his life, then they can definitely continue to say awful things about me going about my day-to-day business. I haven't looked at the comments since. (Although I must admit I do occasionally ask my friend to vet them for me and give me a general feel of them.)

Then Twitter arrived, which was a revelation until accounts began to appear whose sole purpose was to send me abuse. Some days these horrible comments hurt me and some days they didn't, but what upset me more was the realization that there are people in the world who really hate me, despite the fact that they've never met me. People who want to send me abuse and put me down on a regular, day-to-day basis. That's not good for the people-pleaser inside me, the part of me that can't stand anyone not liking me, even people I don't know and would never meet.

Not long ago, I did an in-house chat about mental health with the BBC as part of an awareness-raising week. They asked a group of teenagers what the worst thing was that someone had said to them online. I assumed they would all say something involving their appearance, but I couldn't have been further from the truth. Instead it was, 'Go kill yourself.' I couldn't believe it. Why would you ever want to say that to someone? What could a person have possibly done to you that was that bad? Where had it gone so wrong?

It made me incredibly sad to discover that young people at school were having to deal with abuse like that. When I was at school, I would fall out with friends, then go home for the weekend and everything would be fine again on Monday. Nowadays, these awful, bullying, molesting, harassing conversations are continuing at home and it's impossible to get away from them. They are what you wake up to and go to sleep to. They are part of your psyche. Constantly. For some reason, expressing negative views has become a regular part of online life. Saying something like 'go kill yourself' to someone who is strong and happy in themselves is horrible but it might not have too big an impact on them. However, for someone who's already feeling worthless or questioning whether or not they want to be alive, it could be *fatal*. It makes me go cold to think how I would have reacted to a message like that on one of my darkest days. Would it have just confirmed that ending my life was the right thing to do after all? It doesn't even bear thinking about.

> **Don't listen to these people. Switch off and don't give them the privilege of your time.**

If you do experience abuse online, first of all, I am sorry and it is not fair that people behave in the way they do online. Don't listen to these people. Switch off and don't give them the privilege of your time.

❧

Many psychiatrists have had the experience of being cyber-stalked or defamed or bullied online, and pretty much all of us have treated patients who have been treated in this way. There is no doubt that this behaviour causes mental illness and, in some cases, suicide. Trolling is like daubing graffiti, and the psychology of the trolls I have encountered is in line with the research in the area: they display personality traits of psychopathy, sadism and an inability to empathize with the object of their hate. Trolls use the internet as a way to make themselves feel relevant by abusing people who have what they do not, and they make themselves feel effectual or powerful by provoking or injuring others and disrupting their lives.

It took me a long time to create an Instagram 'profile'. Originally, posting images just felt like yet another thing I had to do, one more thing that was expected of me. I didn't like the idea of sharing more and more of myself, making myself more and more accessible and vulnerable so that people could pick me apart. And the whole selfie thing seemed too self-indulgent. However, when The Saturdays finished and I became a self-employed singer and presenter, it was obvious that I would have to embrace Instagram – it was a brilliant tool for keeping in touch with my fans, sharing new ventures and a way for people to get to know the real me without having to do loads of TV and interviews. And now, it has completely taken over our lives. I look at my Instagram even when I don't care what's on there. I will check it first thing in the morning and last thing at night.

I do feel like I'm stuck between a rock and a hard place with my Instagram posts. I don't want to portray an unrealistic, perfect world on my feed, but I also know that that's what a lot of people want to see. And with so many keyboard warriors out there, all quick to make harsh comments, I'm scared to post anything that will get negative feedback. I don't want someone to tell me that I'm fat, that I'm a bad mum, a bad person, because those are all the things I tell myself already. I don't need to hear my own worst fears externalized and I don't want my horrid, destructive internal voice repeated back to me. We all expose ourselves but also don't want to be targeted.

Of course, not all social media is bad. There has been a mass movement lately that's seen more and more of us trying to be as honest as possible with our followers and, despite my worries about negative feedback, I am trying to do that more, too. There's still a long way to go, but it has already become a brilliant platform for me to share my mental health experiences and to learn about everyone else's too. I get a lot of positive feedback whenever I talk about personal subjects, which spurs me on to do it more often and it means I get to connect to you! So many of us are managing to form amazing support

I don't need to hear my own worst fears externalized.

groups around so many important subjects, which has helped us all feel less isolated. It's reassuring for us all to know that we aren't the only ones to feel this way. But on the flipside, it also allows us to be left exposed to lots of negative accounts and opinions too. I suggest we edit anyone who is a negative force in the community out of our feeds.

But the fact that social media has become the place where people can post the perfect parts of their lives and themselves means that we can constantly compare ourselves to others. And for those of us with low self-esteem (Hi there!) and body-confidence issues, that feeds our biggest fears, insecurities and doubts. This is certainly the issue that affects me the most. Before social media, I could only compare myself to other people in my real life, my imagination, or what I saw on the covers of magazines. Now I have constant proof that everyone else is happier, more successful, prettier, thinner, cooler and more fun than me readily available for me to access on my phone 24/7. I can have confirmation of my own self-hatred whenever I want it.

I do feel that we have to take a lot of the responsibility for how these images make us feel about ourselves and try not to blame others. When I see a picture of a slim girl in a bikini with a big smile on her face, her husband looking at her adoringly and her kids standing perfectly around her, and tell myself that they are all happier than me and my family and that she's better than me because she's thin, that isn't her fault; it's my projection on myself. If I didn't feel so down about myself, I would be able to see that picture for what it is – a normal family who managed to get one good shot out of about a thousand bad ones. And she's probably thin because she has great genes, or works incredibly hard to look that way, or maybe even a combination of both. That woman has nothing to do with me, my life, the way I look or am. Stop comparing.

🄾

Comparisons will only serve to make you unhappy – as Theodore Roosevelt said, 'comparison is the thief of joy'.

We all have to get better at understanding that everything we see on our phone screens has been curated for likes. It's not real. People only project the parts of themselves that they want us to see. It reminds me of my battle with my mental health, always trying to keep up appearances and never showing the real me. It's the same in social media but everyone is doing it and we are caught in a perfect life trap, where no one wants to reveal the truth behind the picture.

I've always been struck by the saying, 'the camera never lies', but I'm not sure that it still stands. I've had friends post a picture looking all loved-up with their other half on a night out, when I know full well that they'd just had a big argument and were having a rubbish time. I do it myself, post a photo saying, 'I'm having a great day', a big smile on my face, when the truth is, I'm having an awful day. I posted a picture of Wayne and me on a night out, not that long ago. There I am in a beautiful, long, flowery dress and there are loads of comments underneath saying how lovely I look. But I felt disgusting. I had sobbed that day about being too ugly to go out.

There is a picture of my bandmate Mollie King and me that sticks in my mind, too. It's from a gig in Ireland where I had a big breakdown. We're walking along with our arms around each other and it looks like a really cute picture of two friends who love each other. However, she was practically holding me up, both physically and mentally. I was at an all-time low, yet if I had posted that picture with a happy caption, you would have taken it at face value. But even knowing the pictures on people's pages don't necessarily tell the truth, I still look at them and believe what I see.

I'm not very good at managing my time on social media. I have tried to stop my phone being the first thing I look at when I open my eyes in the morning and I have also taken full advantage of the 'mute' button to silence the people who make me question myself and bring back bad memories. I have made an effort to follow fewer people with bodies I could never replicate and more people who are living similar lives to me, with kids or the same interests. Or people who inspire me to do things I might never think of doing myself. But social media is a part of my job and a part of all of our lives, so it's hard to switch off from it and relax about not being active online 24/7. There's always that nagging anxiety that my career could end if I didn't post something for 24 hours. It's something we all need to work on. We need to detach ourselves and unplug in order to find a healthy balance between the real us and the social media version of us and our lives.

Remember, be yourself, as everyone else is taken.

Comfort yourself with the knowledge that everyone feels the compare-and-despair trap of social media.

You
are not
alone.

OPEN NOTES

Numerous psychological studies have shown that humans are hard-wired to compare themselves with others. We grow up obsessed with powerful kings and beautiful princesses, and as adults we are equally obsessed with the famous, the rich and the beautiful. In our modern age, we devour stories, pictures and video evidence that we have less than others, and we falsely believe that if only we had what they have, we would be happy. The actual evidence shows that we are seldom satisfied, and that even when we do get what we want, we almost immediately decide that we want and need even more. Everyone from Greek philosophers and Buddha to modern neuroscientists advises us that our only route to happiness lies in accepting that our desires have no limit and that our happiness is much more easily found in accepting who we are and what we have.

Try to enjoy your life in reality. One of the saddest things I have observed in the digital age is people automatically reaching for their mobile phones as their dreams are realized, instead of simply savouring the moment. It seems as though we are becoming dependent on the whole world knowing what a great time we are having, and we are now in danger of spending so much time filming ourselves in paradise that we forget to properly enjoy it while we are there. We all need to enjoy the view rather than sit with our backs to it, hunched over our phones, trying to make sure that everyone we know realizes that we are having a great time while they are not.

Remember, every single one of us is struggling with something. We can only improve ourselves, we can't become someone else, so the only person we should compare ourselves to is a previous version of our own self.

Try not to use your phone as an alarm clock. It's too tempting to check social media through the night and first thing in the morning.

Don't be tempted to write emails or reply to texts before you go to sleep – it will keep your brain alert, especially if you're worried about something.

Try to develop a habit where you turn your phone off before you get into bed. Remember, everything on the internet is there to suck us in, so we need to be vigilant.

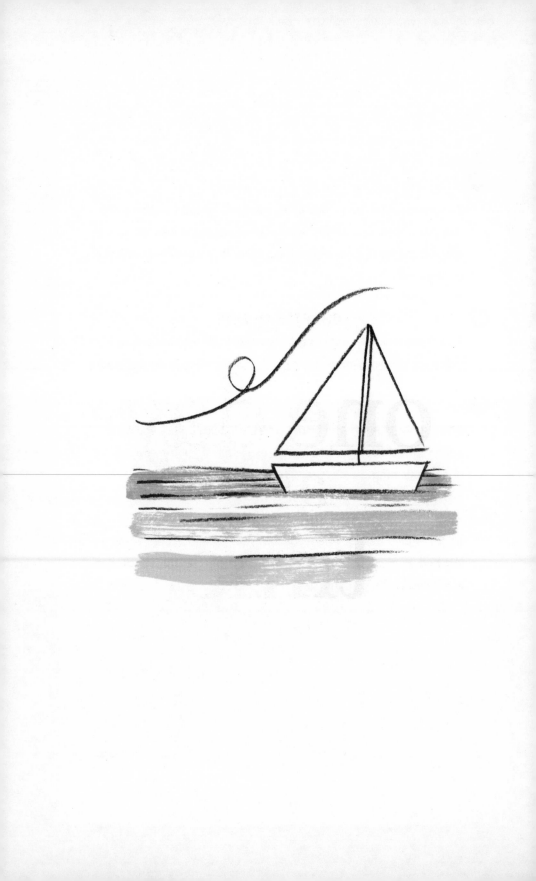

one day at a time

ONE DAY AT A TIME

When I look back over the years, I sometimes wonder how I managed to get through so much of my life without having my illness under control with medicine and treatment. I've got to a stage where I am almost impressed that I could still function when my brain was so fractured and left untreated.

But eventually I did manage to ask for help and I see Mike and Mal as the people who helped to save my life. I'm not convinced that without their help and guidance I'd still be here today, and if I was, I don't think I would have much of a life. I may not see them as often as I used to, but they are still the first people I turn to when I feel my mood slipping. Mike has had to juggle my many different medication trials and I go to Mal when I feel things are piling on top of me in my mind.

I do often feel embarrassed, and even a little selfish, that I only ever talk about myself and keep going over the same issues I've been speaking to them about for the last eight years. There are times when I book in with Mal and by the time I go to see her, I feel I have nothing to say. Then as soon as I sit down and start talking, it all just comes spilling out. Sometimes I leave her office feeling drained and tired, but I always feel better mentally for opening up and letting it all out. I can catastrophize so many things in my head, so saying them out loud helps me gain perspective on whatever they may be.

For me, the two of them – Mal and Mike – come as a pair. I would never rely solely on medication and I could never cope on therapy alone. My medication may not be an absolute cure, as I still have bad days, but I know it will keep me afloat. It gives me a quality of life that I otherwise wouldn't have and stops me from ending up back in hospital. I have learned that my mental health is not something to be messed with or taken for granted.

I always feel better mentally for opening up and letting it all out.

There have been times when I've run out of medication because I haven't noticed I'm running low and haven't ordered my repeat prescription in time. It can take several days for me to really notice a drop in my mood. It usually starts with me wanting to escape back to bed more and hide from the world, then the crying for no specific reason kicks in, followed by the anxiety. And it takes a few weeks to fully recover, like my body is playing catch-up. It still fascinates me that such a small pill can have such an effect on my life. Luckily, my relationship with Mike means that I can check in with him and keep modifying my medication in reaction to my changes in mood. This can be anything from completely changing my antidepressant treatment to adding in a few anti-anxiety pills for a while. You name it, we've probably tried it...

Therapy is equally amazing. I'm lucky to have worked with Mal for so long that she knows me inside out. She knows where most of my anxiety is sourced from and knows now to talk me through and away from my catastrophizing and invasive thoughts. Sometimes I forget to visit her and I realize it's been too long when I start to notice my anxiety has been running away with me, that I've been torturing myself with negative thoughts, or that I've been tearful and avoiding things and situations for a long time and all my old OCD ways have been creeping back in.

If we are born with a vulnerability to worry, as Frankie is, she needs to learn be compassionate to herself and to manage her brain to stop planning and ruminating on negative things.

I try to keep up some form of fitness too. Even after all these years, I still don't actually enjoy it, but I do it because I know I will feel better afterwards. Fitness for me is no good when I'm at the bottom of a dark hole: I have to be able to get myself past that point first. I get frustrated with so many people in the media making it sound so simple – that people with mental health issues should just go and train, then everything will be OK. But that's only possible once you're at a certain level of health. Telling someone who can't even face getting out of bed to wash, get dressed and go to the gym is so counterproductive. It only makes you feel more useless. Yes, exercise really does help, but working out is impossible when you're at rock bottom.

I try to incorporate exercise into my daily routine, but I slip up a lot. What with the boys, work, social life and the days when I'm just not feeling well enough, I'm not very consistent, but I am trying to get better at that. Small things work for me, like walking to places when I can, instead of driving or catching a train. Going out for walks if I don't feel up for a run. I book in classes with friends because then I don't feel I can cancel, and when I'm in a class, I don't feel I can slack off as much.

I have a personal trainer to make me do things when I'm really not in the mood and again I'm booked in, so I have to go. Also when I rope my friends or Wayne into training with me, I feel like I've fitted in a bit of social time to laugh and have a chat as well (when I can actually catch my breath, that is!).

I don't train purely to stabilize my mental health. I'm still someone whose image and weight have a lot to do with my mood, it's something that I think about a lot. And even if I'm not necessarily getting more toned or losing weight, training makes me feel like I'm doing something to keep control of it. And that makes me feel better about the way I look, which in turn improves the way I think.

So much evidence tells us that exercise is good for both the body and the mind. It releases endorphins, the chemicals produced by the body to relieve stress and pain, and also helps with excess adrenaline, which is a result of anxiety. Exercise also helps to increase self-esteem as it gives us a sense of achievement. It is part of learning to take care of ourselves and prioritizing our health.

In truth, there's rarely a day that I don't find hard. But every day I try to wake up with a new perspective and a positive attitude. The great thing about having the kids is that they give me something to get up for. I have to be there for them. Some days are harder than others and occasionally I do sneak up to bed for five minutes to have a moment, but ultimately the boys keep me going. I might not always be the best mum I could be, 24/7, 365 days a year, but I do my absolute best. My children have always been there in the back of my mind during my darker times and they stop me from making rash decisions.

For me, the less downtime I have, the better; but on the flipside, if I'm too busy that also stresses me out. It's a constant battle to find the perfect balance. As someone who's never had the kind of life that could fit into a routine, I now crave one. Now the boys are at school I find that a lot easier, as there are set times when I have to drop them off or be there to pick them up. I tend to exercise straight after drop-off, as that's when I'm at my most productive. If I don't do it then, I often find a way to cancel because my mood dwindles throughout the day. If I have jobs to do, I like to get them done straight after I've exercised, or I go and catch up with some friends. Then, by the time I've gone home and sorted myself out, it's time to get the boys again. The time between pick-up and bedtime is the period I find the hardest. I'm not very good at being at home with nothing to do. The boys are usually tired and just want to chill out, so until dinner time, bath and bed for them, I can find myself slipping into a low mood. This normally leads to me eating everything in sight and then feeling guilty about it.

I'm not very good at being at home with nothing to do. I can find myself slipping into a low mood.

Every morning, I start the day determined to eat well and for the right reasons. I generally do really well all day, but things go wrong in the evening. I don't understand the thinking behind it all – I eat because I'm sad, which then makes me feel even sadder. And fat. And then I eat even more to make myself feel better about feeling fat. It's like I see food as a reward, a treat to myself. I tell myself I have felt low and rubbish all day so I deserve some chocolate to cheer myself up. But of course it doesn't, so I have no idea why I go on doing it, time and time again.

I'm at my best on days when I'm working, which is ironic considering work was once when I was at my most anxious. Now it gives me more purpose and a routine – I'm told when I have to be somewhere, where I'm going and what I have to do. I think I find it reassuring because it's what I have been trained to do and am used to.

Frankie has learned that in order to live with Treatment Resistant Depression, she needs to be prepared to use every tool in her box. She has learned to stop doing what makes it worse (late nights, drinking, overwork, jet lag, not eating properly) and to remind herself to do what makes her feel better (cardio exercise, early nights, talking to people, making the effort to see friends, yoga, meditation, relaxation, good diet).

She has also learned that good compliance with her medication and therapy is crucial, even if she has moments of doubt about whether they are really working. She knows that she cannot guarantee that she will have a good day even if she does every last bit of that, but she also knows that if she does without them, she will have far more bad days.

Remember that every new day is a fresh, new day that has never happened before. And that when it feels like it can never get better, it will.

Nothing in life is totally bad or totally good. So you too, can neither be perfectly happy or perfectly sad. There will be always be room for sadness and happiness to enter your life regardless of what state you currently are in.

I often think it's good we have two feet, as sometimes, what we really need to focus on is putting one foot in front of the other and keep going.

When it feels too tiring,
   which it may do now,
      or may do in the future,
remember asking someone
to help you get back up or
walk alongside you for a while,
   while you get your footing
   is the most powerful and
   important thing to do.

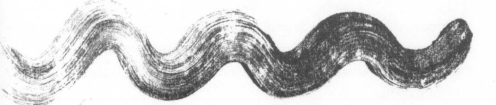

OPEN NOTES

- Remember, avoidance maintains anxiety, so learn to avoid procrastination by setting yourself small goals

- Try to go out at least once a day – even going to the local shop to pick up a pint of milk counts as an achievement

- Each day you should focus on your achievements, no matter how small and reward yourself for it

The psychologist Professor Paul Gilbert writes about how recovery has to revolve around early recognition by the sufferer and being compassionate to ourselves, realizing that depression is part of us, one of our brain systems, but it can't be relied on to be accurate or helpful. Therefore recovery has to focus on recognizing this and using compassion and thinking differently to help ourselves. He reminds us that we don't choose our brains, but it is our responsibility to deal with these vulnerabilities.

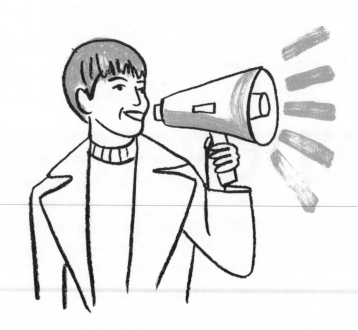

CHAPTER THIRTEEN

speaking
out

SPEAKING OUT

I want to live.

I don't want my life to end now.

I don't want to feel as though I didn't make the most of it.

I don't want to look back and be disappointed.

I will never know what I could have achieved without this illness, but I believe I've done and continue to do the best I can with it.

So I go on as best I can; every day brings a new challenge.

The truth is, I never know how long a good spell is going to last, and I still experience suicidal thoughts. They have always terrified me, because they sneak up on me from nowhere. Most recently, I've had them more at night. I wake up and the intrusive thoughts are sitting there, waiting for me while everyone else is asleep. That's why I always want to let anyone who has lost someone to suicide know that they couldn't have done *anything* to help or prevent it. If I had acted on my thoughts, no one could have helped me.

My suicidal thoughts revolve around two fears, or Negative Automatic Thoughts. One is the feeling that everyone in my life would be better off without me, that the boys and Wayne could go on to find someone better able to handle life and who is more mentally stable. The other is that I'm just tired of this constant battle with myself. I've suffered with this illness pretty much my whole life, and I've done my best, tried my hardest, been the perfect patient, yet here I still am, battling it on a daily basis. The idea of not being here any more is simply a solution to silence my mind and my thoughts.

The truth is, I never know how long a good spell is going to last.

I still have panic attacks and bouts of depression, too. There was a day recently, for example. The whole family was together, we were in the car, the sun was shining, we were all laughing, we'd all had a great day. But by the time we got home, my chest was tight with anxiety, the dark cloud was firmly overhead and I had absolutely no idea why. What I have learnt is to try not to read too much into it or try to get to the bottom of the reason why I feel the way I do. I did try to analyse each panic attack or depression episode and it was wholly counterproductive. I would go around eliminating people and things that I thought were making me feel down, but the truth is, sometimes there isn't a reason. I just have depression and generalized anxiety.

Accept it and move on.

Actually understanding my depression and anxiety has been hugely empowering. The more I understood how and why I feel the way I do, the easier it has become to rationalize and deal with my thoughts.

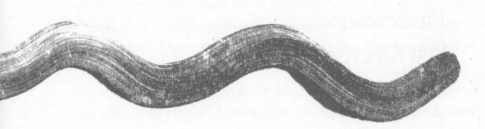

People try to make sense of their depression by referring to what was going on in their lives when it began, but the reality is that a lot of depression has no obvious cause and that it is an illness that simply kicks in at a particular age and follows its own natural course. There may be things that we can do that make it a little better and there is quite a lot that we can do that will only make it worse, but we cannot guarantee that it will go away and stay away.

my panic attacks

I now know that I'm not going to die.
   I will come out on the other side.
   I will be a little shaken.
   But I will also be OK.
      Instead of fighting against it,
      I go with it.
I let it take me over.
   I allow it to engulf every part
   of my body.
I cry uncontrollably.
      I am unable to catch a breath
      and unable to stand.
But I know and trust it will end.
   I know I will be exhausted.
But it will end.
      Panic and sadness can't go on or
      last forever. (And usually end much
      more quickly if I don't fight it.)

Before understanding panic attacks, I would be so terrified by what was happening that I wouldn't be able to breathe. Essentially, I was panicking about having a panic attack. Which is very counterproductive!

If I have that sinking feeling that makes me want to stay in bed and watch mindless TV, I let myself when I can. I only ever allow myself a day at most (any more and I wouldn't leave the house, wash, eat or socialize, so I have to give myself a time limit and some parameters – plus I have two children I need to care for), but sometimes I think it's good to just let yourself feel what you're feeling, lean into it, accept it for what it is, get it out of your system and move on.

My biggest breakthrough on this journey is realizing that I will get through it. And I want you to believe this too. I have been to rock bottom and got myself back up, while also managing to forge a career, friendships, a marriage and raise two children. Nowadays, no matter how low I feel, I know I won't ever be as low as I was when I went into in hospital, because I managed to speak out and ask for help.

> **My biggest breakthrough on this journey is realizing that I will get through it.**

It was such a relief when everyone around me finally knew about my illness – I'd kept it a secret from everyone, including myself, for so long. I was incredibly fearful that people wouldn't understand. I worried that if I told people, they might be scared of me, or judge me and feel that any misstep would lead me to a breakdown. On a professional level, I worried that I wouldn't get jobs because people in my industry might think I was unreliable. (Nowadays, I'd feel that it's more their problem than mine.) When I came out of hospital, it was a huge relief that I didn't have to lie about being OK and hide my illness from the world any more. I wasn't pretending to be another version of myself and, most of all, I didn't have to keep up a performance of pure and constant happiness.

I don't have to live a double life of concealing the showers and constantly being the sunshine.

It is a fact of my working life that I encounter people who will not give me consent to reveal their condition, or its treatment, to their employer. And unfortunately I can perfectly understand why they make that choice. Even though their employment rights are supposedly protected in the UK by the Equality Act, employees are all too aware that they may be subjected to direct and indirect discrimination because of their diagnosis.

Direct discrimination is very obvious – 'You're no use to this company if you can't work 12 hours a day and take calls and emails at the weekend' – whereas indirect discrimination is harder to see, taking forms such as being passed over for promotion. In an industry like Frankie's, while the other members of her band were likely to be supportive, she would have been fearful for any future career options, such as presenting a TV show, because she might be seen as an unreliable proposition because of her history with mental illness.

Now my friends and family understand *both me and my illness*. And although we are one, we have different outlooks; my illness is negative and I try to be positive. They know when to leave me alone but they also know when I might need some more help. They understand that when

I get low, I become withdrawn. I don't go out and I don't reach out to my friends or family for a chat or a catch-up. Now they all realize that my silence means I am having a hard time, so if they haven't heard from me for a few days, they know to check in as my illness is in control. And when they do, it always makes me feel so much better and more like the real me again. Wayne can also tell when I'm having bad days and he instinctively takes over with the kids and leaves me to it. If I cry, he knows that I don't need him to try and fix me, I just need him to hear me out, and then I usually do feel a lot better.

Sometimes, just saying my thoughts out loud to someone else, crying and releasing it all, just helps. Let the pain and fear out. Don't keep it inside.

Most of my friends are people I have known since primary school and their friendships mean a lot to me. I love that no matter where I've been in my career, or the success I've had, they know me for who I truly am. They knew the real Frankie. Before any of that happened. They are the first to bring me back down to earth with a bump. They make me belly laugh like no one else and, most importantly, they have absolutely no judgement, through thick and thin. They know when I'm down and they know when I need space or a catch-up. They know all my deepest, darkest thoughts and I honestly think they are a big part of what has always helped me to stay so grounded over the years.

I am so incredibly close to my sister and we have an amazing friendship. We see things quite differently, which really helps me pull myself back from the brink. She's more of a literal thinker than me and manages to make me see things for what they are. She's also so strong and inspires me to stand up for what I want. I've been lucky to have her to look up to and rely on. The same with my mum and dad, they've learned so much along the way and have become better at opening up and not sweeping things under the rug too. Their generation was so different from ours, things weren't spoken about and they were taught to just get up and get on with it. They've become so much more open and understanding of me and my funny ways. They give me space when I need it, which as a parent now myself, I know is hard to do. They've always let me be who I want to be and they had to let me go at such a young age. My life and career are pretty much down to them allowing me to follow my dreams.

Wayne has been an integral part of my recovery and is still such a huge part of what keeps me going. I appreciate it must be so hard for someone to live with a partner or family member with a mental illness. No two days are the same and it must be so difficult not to take it personally and to live with the inconsistent nature of it, to take each day as it comes. Wayne has had to learn so much. He's great at spurring me on when I need it, but also at giving me a break when I need that too. He'll take the kids out so I can have some time on my own and that can be invaluable. He is my constant sounding board and helps to remind me that my intrusive thoughts just aren't grounded in truth and that reality is so very different.

○

Living with someone who is in a negative spiral is undoubtedly difficult, stressful and exhausting for partners, family and friends. But the people close to someone suffering from mental illness need to be supportive. Encourage the person to seek professional help and try to resist sharing opinions such as 'stay away from medication' as that is a judgement and not necessarily based on fact.

○

Partners and family members shouldn't be afraid of asking for a meeting with treating physicians to help them understand the illness and learn more about how to help the person at home.

Having the boys keeps me going more than anything. I want them to feel loved and heard. They need me and I have to provide for them, be that in the form of love, time, attention or financially. So I have to get up and out of bed for them. That gives me a purpose.

It's taken me years to get my network around me to where it is. It takes time and commitment and courage to be able to open up to everyone around you. To admit you need help and to keep the conversation going. But it's vital to my survival.

That's why it's so important for me to be as open with you as possible. If you are reading this, then there must be a pretty good reason why. I didn't want to write a self-help book because I don't have all the answers, (although I really wish I did!). The only thing that I truly believe in, other than medication, is the power of talking. The importance of being as honest as I can about my thoughts and feelings. Talking about how I feel has literally saved my life, but I know that when you are at the lowest low, you can't see how speaking out would help you. It may be the fear of judgement, or because you don't even understand what you need to say or where to begin. But in order to speak, you don't need to know the answers and you don't need someone else to give them to you, either.

It's. . .

Just understanding that you're not alone.

Just admitting that you're not OK.

Just realizing you cannot do it alone.

All of these small steps can take a huge weight off your shoulders. If you open up to someone when you're at the point where you can't save yourself, they can catch you if you feel you are falling.

The truth is, no one is ever really going to fully understand what's in another person's head, especially if they haven't suffered from mental illness themselves. But they can understand *enough*. Nine times out of ten, I can guarantee that someone you've known for a long time has been suffering in their own way, in silence, and you would never have known.

Not everyone will understand where you're coming from, but they don't judge you and they will be there nonetheless.

I've been very fortunate to be able to have all my treatment privately and I know that not everyone can have that. So make sure you fight for what you need. Take that big step and reach out and ask for help. Even having just one family member or friend that you open up to is better than none. It really is the key to improving your mental health. Just to have one person who you can totally be yourself with, confide all the darkest things to and know that you're not being judged.

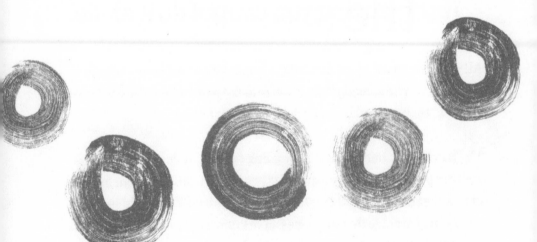

As hard
and scary
as it seems...
You have to find
the strength
to do it.

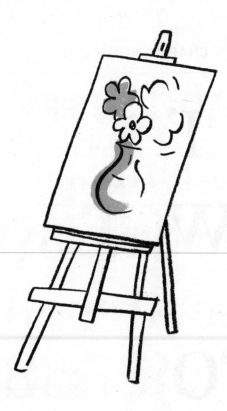

CHAPTER FOURTEEN

I'm a work in progress

I'M A WORK IN PROGRESS

*I have learned to accept that I will
forever be a work in progress.*

On a good day, I have to acknowledge the positives in my situation: I have relationships that are strong and honest, and I have experienced more by the age of 30 than some do in a lifetime. Both the good and the bad.

I am in a position to start the conversation around mental health with a wide audience and to help others to understand themselves more and not feel alone and locked in (which also helps me in turn). It has been so amazing for me to share my story and to feel heard and supported. There is no better feeling than making myself vulnerable and finding out that I am not the only person in the world to ever feel the way I do and to have heard from so many of *you*, that *you* understand, and you've felt it too. Makes me feel as though together we are stronger.

I don't have all the answers. But, what I am doing is trying my hardest every day to lead a full and happy life to the best of my ability. The irony is that writing this book has unsettled my mental health. It shocked me how much I was affected by writing everything down, because

I didn't think I had much of an emotional attachment to my breakdown, especially as it's something I've spoken about quite openly for some time now and that girl – the girl who had a breakdown – feels like a very person different from the person I am now. It was a totally different time in my life and although I wasn't fixed, I have come out on the other side.

The return of my anxiety and my depression getting worse were probably down to the stress of sticking to a deadline and not wanting to let anyone down – my management, my editor, my publisher and you, the reader. I was adamant that I didn't want a ghostwriter as it's such a personal, intimate story. Only I could tell it properly. But I underestimated how hard it would be to write a book. When I spoke to Mal and Mike about the project and the toll it had taken on me, they were both convinced that it was because I was going over a lot of difficult times in my life that I had kept buried under the surface for years and years.

Perhaps subconsciously that is the reason. Perhaps my way of dealing with my past trauma has been to dull it down and put it into a box. I had forgotten a lot of what actually happened and seeing it all there written in my notes made it all very real again, very black and white.

Concentration and memory problems are a normal part of depression and it can take a long time to feel fully recovered after an episode. We do not think that there is permanent damage to most brain functions, but it often scares patients until it is explained that this is a normal part of the illness and that they will recover.

One of the hardest elements of this redisovery has been coming to terms with the fact that I had an eating disorder. I was not aware that it had actually been diagnosed by Mal and Mike, so it was quite a shock to me when they told me. I had to come to terms with the diagnosis through writing about it, and how this eating disorder had been an ally of mine but also a very destructive force in my life.

However, some of the writing about my mental illness has been quite cathartic. Instead of seeing myself as weak because of it, I have realized that I am in fact pretty strong. Anyone who suffers with mental illness on a daily basis and who manages to keep on leading some form of a 'normal' life has to have enormous reserves of strength and energy. Even just getting up and dressed can be a huge achievement, let alone leaving the house, socializing, maintaining friendships, relationships, a career and a family.

Writing about my mental illness has made me realize that I am in fact pretty strong.

I have learned a lot about why I am the way I am and appreciate the journey I have come on. It has made me realize that a lot of my issues come down to control. Something I wasn't wholly aware of before I started writing this book. It is not about me trying to control other people – I am quite laid-back when it comes to others – it is more my *lack* of control in my own life.

Having been in two pop groups where every decision was made for me, I've always wanted to do something from scratch and work it from the ground up all by myself. Truthfully, this book is the first time I've been able to do that in my entire life and it has been hard, but it's felt great. I suppose a lot of it has been taking control of my own life and learning to own it. (There it is again, that controlling 'control' word.)

The truth is, I can't control what happens to me.

I can't control what happens to others.
I can't control how my life will pan out.
   I cannot control other people's
   happiness or wellbeing.
I can't make people safe.
   I can do my best in all these areas.
      But I can't totally control any of it.

Like my fear of flying or going on rides, I have had to give up all the control I have over my safety and put it into the hands of others in order to walk away from my fear. This helps me to understand why I have suffered with an eating disorder, as my food intake was something I could personally control. It is a relief to discover this about myself.

I've always put so much effort into trying to fix other people and myself, and after lots of therapy, I have now realized that that is not my job or my responsibility. These are all things that I suffer with on a daily basis, but I am aware of it now. I can check in with myself and realize that some things need to be left to *just be*.

Having children has definitely helped me to look at life from a different point of view. You realize that they come into the world with no preconceived ideas of how life should be. I love their innocence and how they just see things for what they are, like soap bubbles, or the joy of jumping on a trampoline. The look on their faces in these simple moments are such a brilliant reminder of happiness in the world.

Reminding us to let go and enjoy the small things.
And to let go of the dark.

This does not mean I actually manage to do it all of the time, but it helps. They don't care about the careers Wayne and I have had, how big our house is, how many holidays they get to go on. Instead, they help me to filter out the pressure I put on myself to have more, to earn more. I still have hopes and dreams, but I realize those things are only as important as I make them in my mind. For instance, that new handbag is not going to make me like myself more, make others (or the right people) like me more, it's not going to magically change my life and make me automatically happy.

For me, there's always been that next goal in my life that's going to make me happy and then all my depression will disappear. When I get that number one, I'll feel like my life is complete; if I get that magazine cover, that new job, the big house, the car I've always wanted, lose that extra stone and so on.

The thing is, I've ticked most of my boxes in life, I've managed to reach nearly all my goals, but, of course, I still remain the same. Yes, they come with a great sense of accomplishment, but they don't suddenly make me feel whole. Although I do still torture myself in this way, I am aware of what I'm doing and I do know that there won't be a sudden big change in how I feel. I will always be someone who questions every decision I've ever made. I will always remain a huge 'what if' person – and yes, that's frustrating, but I just can't help it. That pull of self-doubt is just always *too* strong, I can't trust any decisions.

These days, I'm much happier with a smaller life. I still have dreams and goals within my career, I like our life so still hope to keep to a certain level of income, but it's no longer my be-all and end-all. I make

I've ticked most of my boxes in life, I've managed to reach nearly all my goals, but, of course, I still remain the same.

decisions based on my family and my own happiness. I have managed to surround myself with a team that I trust and find inspiring. These are not 'yes' people: I know they will always tell me the truth.

I continue to learn how to say 'no' more. The problem with being a people-pleaser is that I always try to say 'yes', even when it's something that will hurt my mental health. Wayne has always told me it's something that I need to work on. I'm trying to be more selfish, within reason, obviously. I have to weigh things up and try to consider the outcome. For example, if I'm invited to a social event or a work event, I try to decide if I'm anxious about going or whether I know I'll be fine once I'm there, or if it is an environment that I don't actually have to be in and where I don't really need to worry about making the people there happy. If it's a situation that will most likely be fine once I'm there, I'll force myself to go, or I'd never leave the house! If I feel that it's a toxic environment, then I'm starting to find it easier to make my excuses and politely decline. To say 'no'.

I'm constantly learning more about myself and I do feel age has been a great help with that. Also the fact that I now have time to think, as my life is no longer planned out for me, which although scary at first, has meant I love it more. Instead of trying to predict the future all the time and deciding that nothing is going to work out, I just try to take every day as it comes and focus on that. *Try* being the operative word there: it's easier said than done.

For me, my main anxiety these days is my work–life balance. But isn't this the same for most people? The constant guilt of not working enough versus the guilt of working too much. The guilt about how to be 100 per cent present at work and at home.

I have taught myself to accept that I will always be a work in progress. And I need to try to learn to accept that we are all different, that no two lives are the same and one size does definitely not fit all. Of course I'm sad that my happiness levels will never quite reach the heights of others, but I appreciate how lucky I am to have made it this far, and how much fight and passion for life I still have.

Now I see happiness and self-worth as something to work for and not as something that is a given. It is something that I have to take on as my own responsibility, and I have to be willing to work for it as much as I am willing to work hard at my job, my friendships and my family. Others can help me keep up the energy to work towards it, but ultimately it's down to me and only me.

Now, my mental health is out in the open. I can be more open to finding and giving myself the help and love I know I deserve. We all do. So, if you are still living in silence, step out of the dark. Come into the light. It will change your life.

REMEMBER...

We need to accept ourselves, the light and the dark, because we all have a balance of both. We can obsess about our faults and the qualities we lack but if we accept who we are then we will feel less shame. We need to be patient with ourselves and give ourselves time to work on what we need to accept in ourselves.

We need to focus on our strengths and learn to realize that being 'good enough' is not an acknowledgement of failure.

Keep working on it. Recovery could take a lot longer than first thought. And get support. There are lots of free support groups around the country for depression, OCD and other issues.

Recovery does not begin when your symptoms stop. That would be like thinking that your broken leg is back to normal the moment the cast comes off. Your leg will take a long time to regain its full strength and mobility, and it will be many months before you can run your best time after such an injury.

Full recovery means that not only do you have no symptoms of depression, but you are able to sleep normally, think normally, able to absorb stress and upsets in the normal way, able to bounce back from unhappy situations that life inevitably brings with a normal level of resilience, and even perhaps have enough emotional energy left over for helping and supporting others who are struggling. That is a much higher standard of health than simply being out of emotional pain. To get to that place often needs a combination of good medication, good therapy and a range of healthy lifestyle measures, all acting together over six months or more.

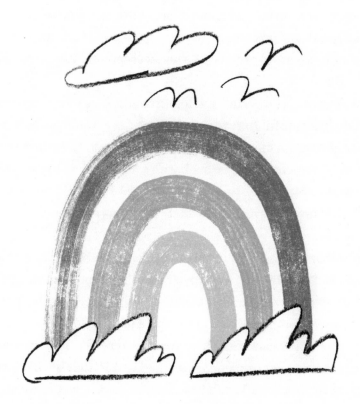

AFTERWORD FROM MIND

Frankie Bridge has been an Ambassador for Mind since 2013. We're incredibly proud of her and grateful for her tireless work to destigmatize mental health and promote a culture of openness. The title she chose for this book is no surprise to us – it's a perfect representation of her values.

Frankie's story is powerful, and told from the heart with tremendous courage. It's painful to read in places, and we would encourage you to take care when moving through her story, and to discuss difficult themes or moments from the book with someone close to you (you can also speak to Mind – see page 243 for details). How did it feel when you read this? Have you ever felt like that? What works for you?

Open is, in many ways, a story about power. In the beginning, Frankie doesn't feel like she has any power over her experiences, and that difficult thoughts and feelings have control over her life. The first time she accesses therapy, she struggles with a new sense of loss. Realizing you're struggling can affect how you see yourself, though of course it's important to get the support you need – and that is what Frankie is urging us to accept. We all have mental health, just as we all have physical health; sometimes it is good, sometimes it is less so.

Most of us won't share Frankie's particular life experiences – not many of us are in successful pop bands, or have access to some of the options available for getting help with our mental health. But in many ways, Frankie's story is also universal – there are high points, low points, personal challenges and changing relationships. She shares her emotional responses to each experience with bravery and candour. The healthcare professionals she sees offer her one explanation for her experiences, but there is another power story in play here too; each time life gets tough, Frankie learns a little more about herself, and what she needs to cope.

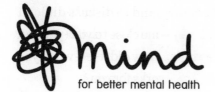

HELP AND SUPPORT

Like Frankie, we want everyone experiencing a mental health problem to get support and respect.

To learn more about mental health, including the different models, or ways of thinking about it, as well as information about different experiences, treatments and support options available, go to www.mind.org.uk/information-support/

You can also contact Mind's InfoLine, where our team provides information on a range of topics including:
- Types of mental health problems
- Where to get help
- Medication, talking therapies, and other treatments
- Advocacy

We will look for details of help and support in your own area.

CONTACT US

Our lines are open 9am to 6pm,
Monday to Friday (except for bank holidays).
0300 123 3393
info@mind.org.uk
Text: 86463

Mind Infoline
PO Box 75225, London E15 9FS

Our local Mind services support hundreds of thousands of people across England and Wales every year. Each local Mind is unique. They understand the needs of their community and they tailor their services to match. The services include talking therapies, crisis helplines, drop-in centres, employment and training schemes, counselling and befriending. Contact yours to see how they can help you. You can find your local Mind on our website at www.mind.org.uk/information-support/local-minds/

GLOSSARY

Acceptance and Commitment Therapy (ACT) is a type of psychotherapy that aims to help people open up to, and accept, emotions as appropriate responses to certain situations.

anhedonia The inability to feel pleasure, this is a common symptom of depression and other mental health disorders.

anorexia People who have anorexia nervosa, commonly referred to as anorexia, try to keep their weight low by restricting food and/or over-exercising. They often behave in a ritualized way around food and have a distorted image of their bodies. This is a life-threatening illness, with the highest mortality rate of any psychiatric disorder. It is most common in young women, but men and women of any age can suffer from it.

Beck Depression Inventory (BDI) This is a multiple-choice psychometric test that people complete by assigning a score to 21 key symptoms of depression, including mood, sense of failure, guilt, self-dislike, suicidal thoughts, crying, social withdrawal, indecisiveness, body image change, insomnia, loss of appetite and loss of libido. It is widely used to measure the severity of depression.

binge eating disorder Most sufferers regularly lose control of eating, consuming very large amounts of food in a short time, frequently secretly or while alone. Binges are often planned ahead and followed by feelings of guilt.

bipolar disorder Previously known as manic depression, this is a mental health condition where people have moods that go from one extreme to the other, with episodes of significantly elevated mood (manic or hypomanic) followed by feeling very low and lethargic (depression). Each extreme episode of bipolar disorder can last several weeks or even months.

bulimia nervosa Known simply as bulimia, this is characterized by sufferers overeating, as with binge eating disorder, but then taking compensatory action such as vomiting, using laxatives or diuretics, fasting or doing excessive amounts of exercise.

Cognitive Behavioural Therapy (CBT) Widely practised, this is one of the most effective forms of psychotherapy. It is a talking therapy that focuses on changing the way people think and behave as a way of coping and dealing with different mental health problems.

Dialectical Behavioural Therapy (DBT) Developed in the 1980s by psychologist Marsha M Linehan, DBT is a type of Cognitive Behavioural Therapy that aims to identify and change negative thinking patterns.

Generalized Anxiety Disorder (GAD) A long-term condition, GAD causes people to feel anxiety about a broad range of situations and conditions. They tend to catastrophize possible end results, magnifying the dangers that might occur and underestimating their ability to cope.

Negative Automatic Thoughts (NATs) make sufferers put a negative interpretation on what they think is happening to them, ignoring positive or neutral information. Examples of NATs include catastrophizing (always picturing the worst possible outcome), over-generalizing (one thing going wrong means everything is going to go wrong), mind reading (assuming that people know what the sufferer is thinking and feeling) and personalizing (something that goes wrong confirms that the sufferer is worthless).

Obsessive Compulsive Disorder (OCD) Usually beginning in early adulthood, OCD is a common mental health condition, where a person has obsessive fears or thoughts and compulsive behaviours in response to these. OCD can be treated by Exposure and Response Prevention, whereby the person is exposed to their fear and then prevented from using a compulsion to neutralize it. In the short term, this treatment causes the person's anxiety to increase but the brain soon realizes that there is no real threat.

orthorexia nervosa An obsession with eating only foods that the sufferer believes to be 'pure' or 'healthy', the symptoms of orthorexia include eating very little food, exercising too much, spending a disproportionate amount of time obsessing about food and becoming preoccupied with body shape.

Post-Traumatic Stress Disorder (PTSD) First observed in soldiers and given a number of names, such as shell shock, PTSD is an anxiety disorder that is caused by experiencing or witnessing a very distressing or frightening event or events.

Prozac A type of SSRI, this is often used to treat depression, Obsessive Compulsive Disorder and bulimia. It tends to have fewer side effects than other forms of antidepressant.

SNRIs (serotonin and norepinephrine re-uptake inhibitors) These antidepressants are similar to, but designed to be more effective than, SSRIs (see below), and some people seem to respond to them better.

SSRIs (selective serotonin re-uptake inhibitors) Often the first choice, as they have fewer side effects than most other types of antidepressant, these are mainly prescribed to treat depression, particularly persistent or severe cases, often in combination with a talking therapy. They are thought to increase serotonin levels in the brain.

Repetitive transcranial magnetic stimulation (rTMS) is a non-invasive type of brain stimulation therapy in which a magnetic field is targeted at specific areas of the brain to treat depression and anxiety.

INDEX

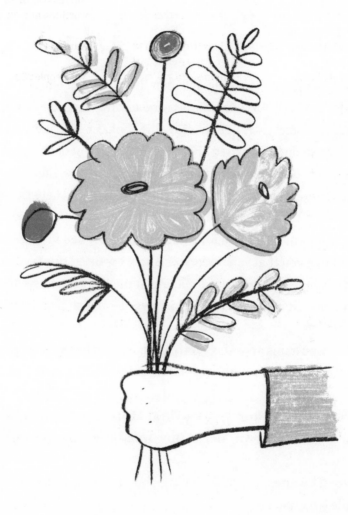

FRANKIE'S ACKNOWLEDGEMENTS

This book is a prime example of 'when life gives you lemons, make lemonade'. Taking a horrible situation and finding the good in it. If you had asked me a few years ago to write this book, I would have said no. I would have been too worried about the judgement of opening up and being honest about some of the most difficult times of my life. However, being surrounded by the right people changed that, and here we are...

Romilly Morgan, thank you for totally getting my vision. I knew the moment I met you that you understood how I wanted this book to be. You've been sensitive but also amazing at pushing me to go deeper. Thank you for giving me confidence in myself every step of the way.

Charlotte Abrahams and Alex Stetter, you have to be the most patient women ever! Putting up with my email-avoiding and my awful spelling.

Thank you to Jack Storey, Jaz Bahra, Marianne Laidlow, Kevin Hawkins, Caroline Brown, Megan Brown and everyone at Octopus.

Stephanie Thwaites, you took a chance on me, put my idea out there and made it happen.

Meryl Hoffman, this was all your idea. You always believe in me, even when I don't. You push me to do things out of my comfort zone and you are always my biggest cheerleader. Your excitement and drive is infectious. I love working with you. I've written a book!

Josh Byrne, thanks for constantly repeating emails you know I'm avoiding and making me laugh.

Mollie, Una, Vanessa and Rochelle, thank you for holding the fort together while I couldn't. Peter, you gave me the time and understanding I needed for recovery, which I know must have been difficult.

Mal, Mike and MeeMee, you literally saved my life. And for that I will be forever grateful. Thank you for helping me to help others.

Friends, for sticking around and putting up with my weirdness and my bouts of disappearance. The belly laughs we have help more than you will ever know. I can always be myself with you.

Mum and Dad, sorry it took me so long to be honest with you about my illness. You've supported me through this whole madness I call my life. I have everything to thank you for. If it wasn't for you guys believing in me from the start and making the brave decision to let me go on and live my dream, I wouldn't be where I am today. So many of my life boxes are ticked because of you, while making sure my feet stay firmly on the ground! I really hope this book helps you to release any misplaced guilt and realize that it's just the way I am. I probably don't say it enough, I love you and thank you.

Tor, you've always been my best friend and the voice of reason. You help to let out my fun side and see the lighter side of life. At the same time, you make sure I never get too big for my boots! I love that you're my someone who's always there no matter what, no questions asked. I'm so lucky to have a sister like you. I'm so glad that I get to repay you with all the fun parts of my job...as you say.

Wayne, thanks for sticking by me through it all. I know this has often been the hardest for you. The person who is closest to it all day-to-day and has to pick up the pieces. You always do your best to understand. You stuck by me at a point in the beginning when you could have easily walked away. You are a massive part of my recovery then and now and I will forever be grateful for that. You've given me all I wanted from life, my own little family. Thank you for loving me regardless of my crazy.

Parker and Carter, you are my reason for living. I knew I wanted you before I'd even had you and you were my reason to take the step towards recovery. Every day I wake up and start all over again for you. You inspire me to see the joy in life. I will continue to raise mental health awareness, so that you can live a life without stigma. I hope you always feel able to be open and honest. Love you more than the world.